Power Living

Power Living

Everybody's Health and Diet Book

Ira Kellman
with
Jonita Mullins

Treasure House

An Imprint of

Destiny Image® Publishers, Inc.

P.O. Box 310

Shippensburg, PA 17257-0310

"For where your treasure is
there will your heart be also." Matthew 6:21

ISBN 1-56043-792-8

For Worldwide Distribution
Printed in the U.S.A.

Treasure House books are available through these fine distributors outside the United States:

Christian Growth, Inc.
Jalan Kilang-Timor, Singapore 0315

Rhema Ministries Trading
Randburg, South Africa

Salvation Book Centre
Petaling, Jaya, Malaysia

Successful Christian Living
Capetown, Rep. of South Africa

Vine Christian Centre
Mid Glamorgan, Wales, United Kingdom

Vision Resources
Ponsonby, Auckland, New Zealand

WA Buchanan Company
Geebung, Queensland, Australia

Word Alive
Niverville, Manitoba, Canada

Inside the U.S., call toll free to order:

1-800-722-6774

Or reach us on the Internet: **http://www.reapernet.com**

Dedication

This book is dedicated to all those individuals who long to be healthy and whole, and who are willing to become the very best they can be.

Contents

Spiritual

Foreword

I'm glad to finally see a powerful book on exercise, diet, and health that doesn't ignore the emotional, mental, and spiritual needs of people. Ira has produced an instructional book that gently leads people with good hearts but lazy legs into developing a healthy life style, exercising the spirit, mind, and body.

With many years of traveling around the country, I've had numerous opportunities to observe people in churches and social gatherings. Most everyone stands around the buffet table drinking coffee (with cream and sugar!) and eating cookies and donuts after enjoying an inspiring sermon, stimulating lecture, or wonderful concert or film. They have filled themselves up spiritually and mentally, but are unaware or unconcerned about how they fill themselves up physically.

This book is loaded with powerful insights into the way we function and how we can improve our quality of life. Ira is right when he says, "We truly live when we are whole people, growing and learning and becoming in every area of our lives." His book is a must-read for anyone who wants to be whole and healthy in every way.

Kim Alexis, supermodel

Preface

I don't know anyone who doesn't want to live their lives to the fullest measure possible. We all want to look good, feel good, and do good. Yet this desire is not so easily accomplished. That's why I have shared my thoughts and experiences in this book dedicated to everyone who wants to be a healthy and whole individual.

We are not simply physical beings. We are people with a mind, heart, and spirit that needs to be nurtured and nourished. To be healthy and whole, we must care for the whole person—including body, mind, emotions, and spirit. Through the pages of this book, I want to take you on a journey of discovery into ways to bring health and happiness to the whole you.

So grab a pencil and notebook and prepare to learn about yourself. In this journey of learning, I believe you'll find a wonderful, whole, happy individual inside just waiting to be recognized. You can find your full potential and become the person you want to be.

Mental

Chapter 1

You Are What You Think

Life is a mirror and will reflect back to the thinker what he thinks into it.

—Ernest Holmes

So much has been written about health and dieting—is there anything new we could say on the subject? With all the diet books, diet programs, and diet drinks on the market, you'd think we would all be happy, healthy, and *thin* by now. But we aren't. It's a well-known fact that many people—young and old, male and female, rich and poor—struggle with their weight, their health, and their self-esteem.

As an evangelist, I travel to churches in both the United States and Europe. I've seen people who are struggling for balance and control in their lives. I've talked with them and counseled with them about the health problems they were creating for themselves.

I'm convinced that dieting has very little to do with food. Oh, sure, we need to watch what we eat; that's common sense. (We'll deal with that issue in a later chapter.) But dieting is just as much a matter of the mind and the spirit.

Very few diet books address the soul and spirit of man; yet we are spirit beings. Whatever affects our bodies, first affects our minds, hearts, wills, emotions, and spirits. We cannot separate one part of us from another. To try to lose weight by only counting calories is to miss the greater challenge of becoming a *whole* person, not simply a *thin* person.

Weight problems nearly always begin in the mind. In fact, most of our problems begin there. Therefore, the solutions to these problems also begin in the mind. Proverbs 23:7a tells us how important our thoughts and beliefs are to our character and actions. It says, "For as he thinketh in his heart, so is he."

What you think is far more important than what you eat. I'm sure you've heard the expression, "You are what you eat." That may be true, but it is even more true that you are what you think because you become what you think in the process of time.

Beliefs Are Important

Marcie grew up believing she wasn't pretty. She had to wear glasses and by the time she was in the sixth grade she was taller than everyone else in her class. She was painfully self-conscious of her height and appearance.

Because of her belief, which was reinforced by the teasing of thoughtless children, Marcie convinced herself that she could never be attractive. Food became her companion, her solace. She gained weight gradually but steadily, always thinking that it didn't matter anyway. Nature had given her that body and there was no hope of anything different.

When she became a Christian after graduating from high school, Marcie began to learn more about her worth as a person. She found out that all her negative thoughts were not the result of how she looked, but the cause of how she looked. If she could change her thoughts, then she could change her behavior; and that would bring a change in her appearance. She put her new beliefs to work and in time lost 30 pounds.

There is a definite relationship between our beliefs about our bodies and the appearance of our bodies. Most doctors agree that people with weight problems or addictions have a negative self-image. The following simple formula illustrates how our beliefs affect every other part of our lives.

Belief + Behavior = Results

Remember, Proverbs 23:7a says, "For as he thinketh in his heart, so is he." What you believe about yourself will determine every action you take. If you believe you are fat, for example, your body will comply with that belief. You will be fat. Others might not see you as fat, but you will. When you look in the mirror, that is what you will see.

If you should lose weight, but not lose the belief that you are fat, your weight loss probably won't last. Your belief will influence your behavior and the same habits and eating patterns that first created the weight problem will remain as long as the faulty belief is unchanged.

What Do You Think About You?

You must think positive, healthy thoughts if you wish to become a positive, healthy person. Changes on the outside occur only after changes on the inside have taken place. You need to identify the wrong thoughts and beliefs that are sabotaging your own happiness and health. Then you must change those thoughts and beliefs.

So many people appear as if they don't care *about* themselves because they don't care *for* themselves. They don't like themselves. They spend a great amount of time wishing they were someone else. They feel ugly and unloved because they think ugly, unloving thoughts.

Proverbs 11:17 says, "The merciful man doeth good to his own soul: but he that is cruel troubleth his own flesh." A great many people trouble themselves with condemnation, rejection, hatred, self-pity, and other negative, destructive thoughts. They fall into bad habits and patterns of behavior as a result of those thoughts. These people are cruel to their flesh by feeding themselves first the wrong thoughts, then the wrong actions, and finally the wrong food.

We all want to be able to look in the mirror and feel good about ourselves. But how can that happen if the first thought that comes to our minds when we look in the mirror is, "Oh, yuk"? We say what we think, and our actions and reactions eventually reflect our attitude toward ourselves.

Do you ever hear yourself saying such things as, "I'm fat; I'm stupid; I'm not coordinated; I'm shy"? We may think we don't mean those things when we say them. They are simply remarks meant to show that we aren't arrogant or vain. However, they are still put-downs. If we listen to them long enough, we begin to fulfill them. Those words are the subtle signs of what we are thinking about ourselves.

Proverbs 12:25 says, "Heaviness in the heart of man maketh it stoop: but a good word maketh it glad." If you have ever told yourself, "You're no good; you can't change; you've been on every diet known to man and you're still overweight," then you are pulling yourself down. You are creating the weights that create the weight problem of the other problems of phobias, failures, and addictions.

We become what we think just as we become what we eat. Therefore, to change what we are, we must change what we think. In order to do that, we must identify what we think about ourselves.

Are we sabotaging our own efforts at being healthy and happy by thinking negative, hurtful thoughts? Are we harboring hurts from the past—resentments and frustration, fears and disappointment, anger and bitterness?

Often the hurts of our childhood are buried deep within our subconscious mind. We can repress these memories and seem to forget them. But they are still there, working inside us. We would probably be surprised at how much these past pains affect our present thoughts and actions.

Repressed memories, anger, bitterness, resentment, and frustration are not healthy. They don't promote the qualities that we must have in our lives if we are to be successful individuals. These are the things that must be changed.

Take some time now to examine your thinking. I can't begin to list all of the complexes, fears, pains, and doubts that people deal with every day. Each individual faces a unique set of factors that play a part in what he or she thinks. Hopefully these general things I've mentioned have shed light on your mind and the thoughts that lie there. If you can recognize the problem areas in your thinking, you can begin to find the solutions.

The Mind Is Not a Vacuum

The solution to destructive thinking is not to merely say, "Well, I'll just stop thinking those awful thoughts." That is not enough. You can't shut down your brain and think nothing.

Unless you are in a coma right at this moment (in which case you wouldn't be reading this book), you *are* thinking. Also, even if you were in a coma, your subconscious mind would still be thinking. You think something all the time, in everything you do.

If you intend to get rid of the negative thoughts, you must replace them with positive ones. Your mind is not a vacuum. Empty it of one thought and another one will rush in to fill the vacant spot. Your job is to fill the vacancy with something good. Here are some steps you can take to change your thoughts and beliefs.

First, face the facts. Know what is happening in your mind. Look squarely at everything that has happened in your life that created those negative beliefs about yourself. If you were hurt by someone else, or if you are hurting yourself with destructive thoughts, acknowledge it. Then identify the problem areas by looking at them as honestly as you can.

Next, evaluate your beliefs and thoughts. Which critical thoughts are justified and which are blown out of proportion? Put your thoughts in the proper perspective. Recognize the lies you have been telling yourself or that perhaps others have been telling you.

Then decide what you want to be. Remember, what you think is what you become. If you want to change your thinking, you must know the good thoughts you want to think. Write down the results that you seek in your life. Establish goals and develop an image in your mind of the type of person you intend to become. Then you can focus your thoughts in that direction.

It's a matter of deciding what you want to become. It sounds so simple, yet many people wander through life never knowing where they want to go. They have no plans for tomorrow, or next year, or even ten years from now. Others do have goals, but those goals are so vague and uncertain that they create frustration rather than results.

If you start a diet without a weight-loss goal in mind, you will always be on a diet because you will never reach a goal. Constant dieting is futile and frustrating—and so is trying to rid yourself of negative thoughts without having something better to replace them with.

"For as he thinketh in his heart, so is he." Think on what you want to become. Your goals don't have to be great and earth-shattering. They can be simple, such as, "I want to look good in that suit. I want to fit into those jeans. I want to look good and feel good!"

Think about the things that will bring you victory in reaching your goal. Tell yourself, "I'm changing. I'm growing. I'm becoming the person I want to be." Create new thought patterns and new beliefs about yourself. It may take time, but it will bring results—if you start now.

Everything in life seems to go better when you feel good about yourself. Even when difficulties and tragedies come (for they come to all of us), you can handle them much better if you have a positive belief system working on your side. So watch what you feed your mind. Be careful of the thoughts you let dwell there. Change your thinking to change your life.

What If I Can't Change?

Right about now you might be thinking, "Sure, that sounds good, but what if I can't change? I've been like this all my life. I can't suddenly become a different person."

What kind of thoughts are those? They're self-defeating thoughts, the very ones that need to be changed. Fear of change is one of the major stumbling blocks people face in overcoming a life-controlling problem such as overeating, alcoholism, or some other addiction. No matter how miserable we might be in our present condition, it often seems preferable to the unknown, the pain, and the hard work of change.

As a result we invent excuses for not trying. Here are some excuses people use to justify not changing. See if they sound familiar to you.

1. It's too difficult to change.

Most of the worthwhile things people have done in this world were at first declared impossible. So it's never too hard to change if you take it slowly, one step at a time. You also need to work with an understanding of yourself and what you should change. You must find the motivation to change by setting some realistic, yet challenging and exciting goals.

It takes a certain daring to want to change and to overcome the fear of changing. It requires seeing yourself moving into a new role just as an actor would. Actors do what they can to conform to their roles. It might be gaining or losing weight, changing their hair color, or spending hours in make-up. The key is getting the inspiration to rise to that role.

How much do you want a new you? Are you willing to work at it? You can win if you believe you can.

You simply have to want the change more than you want the security of staying the same.

2. I don't have self-control.

You do have self-control; you simply must exercise it. Self-control, like a muscle, grows with use. You begin to build your self-control in small ways. Saying "no" to a second helping at dinner may be one simple way to begin controlling your eating habits. Once you have mastered that, you can move on to other challenges.

No one exhibits perfect self-control all the time. We all have our moments of weakness and failure. If you slip once or twice or more, that doesn't mean you don't have self-control.

Don't give up after a failure either. Someone once said, "You are never a failure if you get up one more time than you fall." Every step you take in gaining control over your thoughts, your behaviors, and your life is worth the effort. Exercise the muscle of self-control and you will become a strong, healthy person.

3. I'll never be able to change because I've failed so many times in the past.

No matter what your past has been, you can be free from it. All you need is plenty of time, understanding, and patience. The only hold the past has on today is in your mind. It doesn't matter how many times you might have failed in the past. What matters is what you are trying to do right now, in the present.

Abraham Lincoln failed at just about everything he attempted, until he ran for President. But he never gave up and because he persisted, became one of the greatest men in history. Read the biography of any successful individual and you will almost certainly find that he or she had many failures, disappointments, and obstacles to overcome. If you have failed in the past, then you are in very good company.

Learn the lessons of your mistakes and then forget the mistakes. Begin again right now. You can change today no matter what you did yesterday.

4. I don't like to be uncomfortable, and change makes me uncomfortable.

I won't promise that you'll never be uncomfortable as you begin to change things in your life. But when exercised slowly, discipline builds up your tolerance for any discomfort or pain changing may cause you.

You don't have to become a completely new person overnight. You didn't get to be the way you are in one 24-hour time period. You won't change the way you are in that amount of time either. Look at change as a long-range goal. It is something you will be doing for the rest of your life if you are healthy and determined to keep growing, learning, and becoming.

Besides, the results of a happier, healthier you far outweigh the pain of change. Keep your eye on the goal. Stay focused on what you are becoming, not on what you are leaving behind. With time, you'll wonder why you ever wanted to stay the way you were, and you won't even remember the pain.

5. I don't want to face my beliefs and behaviors.

Desire is the first step to change. If you don't want to face yourself honestly, chances are you will find any excuse not to do so. The question you must ask yourself is this: "Am I content to be the way I am right now for the rest of my life?" If the answer is no, then you do have the desire to change.

Let that desire fuel your determination to face yourself honestly. You must deal with who you are, what you think, and how you behave. You won't find yourself to be a terrible person. No, you are human and we humans all have things we must deal with in our lives. We all have our faults, failings, and simple misunderstandings. Don't be afraid of what you might find.

When you face the real you, then you will be in a much stronger position to develop a better you. If you want to make the best of yourself, then you do want to face your beliefs and behaviors—and you can.

6. I can't think right because of what happened in my past.

As I said before, the past is past. It's gone. The only connection the past has to the present is through our memories. Thoughts about the past are like chains that keep us bound to the people and problems we have known. These people and problems may have long since passed out of our lives, but if we keep them alive in our minds, they will continue to hurt and hinder us.

If the negative thoughts that undermine your progress are the results of hurts and struggles from your past, you must face that past. Then you must bury it. Hold a funeral for it if you have to, but get it behind you and move on with your life. Never let your yesterdays use up your todays.

Don't let old decisions and experiences keep you from being healthy and disciplined today. Forgive those who need forgiveness, including yourself. Then forget the past by refusing to let it linger in your memory. You can choose a new way of thinking and of living.

7. I am destined to be just like my parents.

Certainly our parents have a tremendous influence upon our lives. The traits we inherit through our genes are things over which we have little choice or control. But we shouldn't use our parents as an excuse not to change or become better.

I know of a woman who says it is her mother's fault that she weighs more than 300 pounds. "My mother made me clean my plate at every meal," she says. "That's why I can't stop eating now." No doubt her mother's influence was a strong force in this woman's life. But she has made that influence an excuse to eat. Her mother isn't making her eat now; the choice to eat or not is hers alone.

You may have learned some bad habits or developed some negative thinking patterns while growing up, but you can change. Replace the bad habits with good ones. Replace the negative thoughts with positive ones. You can train yourself to be the person you want to be.

8. I don't want to give up my present thoughts or habits.

Ralph Waldo Emerson wrote, "Men wish to be saved from the mischief of their vices, but not from their vices." That sums us all up fairly well, I think. We want to be free of the problems our thoughts and habits cause us, but not necessarily from the thoughts and habits. It's much more difficult to be free of those. We don't want to give up our self-pity or the chocolate cake that self-pity caused us to eat.

Ask yourself, "Is this how I want to spend the rest of my life? Will I be controlled by negative thinking and destructive behavior, or will I control my thoughts and my actions?" The decision is yours.

Don't look at change as having to give up something. Look upon change as gaining something better. Seek your freedom from controlling thoughts, substances, and actions. Then you will be free to choose the things that you truly enjoy and that are beneficial to you.

Put Away Childish Things

Much of what we must overcome to change our thinking is related to the past. We are the products of all that happened to us throughout our lives.

There are many people who absolutely hate cats because they were scratched by a cat when they were young. It doesn't matter to them that some cats (such as my own cat, King) are gentle and well-behaved and would never deliberately scratch anyone. These people hate cats—period. One bad experience left a very lasting impression on their minds.

I know people who don't like to eat vegetables simply because they were forced to do so as children. People who have a prejudice against vegetables won't have very healthy eating patterns. Thus a childhood memory creates problems for an adult body.

"I don't like spinach," they will say, when perhaps they haven't even tried to eat spinach since they were eight years old and it lay green and slimy on their plate. The reactions of an 8-year-old to spinach should hardly be the basis of a decision made by a 30-year-old adult. But too often it is. So what if 20 years ago you didn't like spinach? It's today now. Isn't it time to put away some of those childish thoughts and behaviors?

The apostle Paul wrote in First Corinthians 13:11,"When I was a child, I spake as a child, I understood as a child, I thought as a child: but when I became a man, I put away childish things." We cannot change the things that have happened to us in the past; we can only change how we deal with them in the present. Sometimes what we need to do is put away childish, or childhood, things.

Of course, there are pains and problems from the past that are much more serious than cats and spinach. I don't mean to say that everything that happened to us as children was trivial. I recognize that many people endured abuse, rejection, disabilities, sorrows, and many other hurtful things as they were growing up. The problems are very real, but the solution is not to give in to those things. We must overcome them. We must put those things away.

"But I can't forget," some people say. "I can't put this behind me. The scars run too deep." A scar is a sign that a wound has healed. Scars do not run deep; only wounds do. If you are dealing with a wound rather than a scar, then perhaps the wound was never allowed to heal.

Your mother probably told you that if you kept pulling off the bandage to look at the scratch, it would never heal. The same is true for emotional and mental wounds. If you replay the pain over and over again, you continually reinflict the wound. It will never heal that way.

You must put it away. Only then will your thoughts become healthy and positive. Only then will you be ready to change and develop into the positive, healthy person you want to be and were meant to be.

Think Healthy

By now you know that I firmly agree with Solomon's assessment of the importance of our thoughts. "For as he thinketh in his heart, so is he" (Prov. 23:7a). If you think healthy, then you will be healthy. If you think thoughts of healing, forgiveness, love, faith, confidence, and hope, then you will have all those things in your life.

Healthy thinking can mean the difference between living a victorious "on top of the world" life and living a mediocre "just getting by" life. It affects every choice, every action, and every reaction we make.

My co-writer and I were driving to the library one day to do some research for this book. We ran into a traffic snarl because of road construction. While we were sitting at a stop light, a woman pulled up beside us. She had the most frustrated look on her face. I could tell just by looking at her that she wasn't thinking healthy thoughts.

She impatiently pulled into the intersection, but couldn't get through because of the road equipment. So there she sat, right in the middle of the intersection. She created even more traffic problems because of her impatience and unclear thinking, and she nearly collided with the tar machine!

We couldn't get through the intersection because of her car, so I simply backed up a little and pulled into a parking lot. Then we turned and went around the block, leaving the frustration and traffic problems behind. There was no hassle, no waiting, and no messy tar to clean off my car. That was healthy thinking.

When you begin to think in healthy, positive ways, you will find yourself leaving many of the old ways and thoughts behind. There won't be any room in your life for frustration, anger, bitterness, or regret. These will be buried in the past where they should be. You'll be moving on into a better life style and finding a healthier you.

Thinking healthy is not for an hour, a day, or a week. It must be developed as a way of life. So remember these points for thinking healthy and being healthy.

1. Health and fitness begin in your mind and with your attitudes.

Your thoughts and beliefs are the most important factors in living life to the fullest. If your thoughts are healthy, you will be healthy.

2. Your beliefs determine your behavior.

You act upon what you believe about yourself and about the world around you. It doesn't matter nearly as much what others think of you as what you think about yourself. Any effort to change a harmful habit must be accompanied with a change in the beliefs that caused that habit.

3. Your past is not in control of you.

Everyone has had a share of unhappiness, but healthy people do not dwell on it. Don't keep looking back with sadness or guilt. Say to yourself, "I did the best I could at the time," and then go on living in the present.

4. Replace negative thoughts and behavior patterns with positive ones.

Start the day with a healthy therapy: Bible study, exercise, peaceful or upbeat music. Always be busy working on problems, looking for solutions, finding answers. Accentuate the positive in everything you think, say, and do. Help those who are less fortunate than yourself.

5. Like who you are.

Never become complacent, but don't compare yourself with others either. Enjoy your life. Fill it with the things that are good for you and that give you pleasure. Accept yourself even as you work to improve yourself. Set lifelong goals and you will stay youthful and healthy with an enduring zest for living.

Healing of a sickness or injury can come as an instantaneous miracle, but health is the practice of a lifetime. Changing our thinking to be positive and healthy probably won't happen overnight. We must work at it day by day.

Think of it as a football game. A football team doesn't try to score a touchdown with every play. Their short-range goal is to get the first down, and they have four tries to do that. If they can gain the first downs, they can eventually reach the goal line and score. They want to travel down the field without losing ground through penalties or quarterback sacks.

Likewise, in your efforts to change and grow, keep moving forward. Don't give up the ground you've gained by penalizing yourself with doubts, fears, or other negative thoughts. You can be a winner in this game.

An old Arabian proverb says, "He who has health, has hope; and he who has hope, has everything." Health is much more than just a body that is fit and trim. It involves every part of you—body, spirit, and soul. Healthy thoughts create healthy attitudes and beliefs; they inspire healthy behaviors and habits, and they in turn result in a healthy life. You are what you think!

Chapter 2

The Words You Eat

The soul, like the body, lives by what it feeds on.

—Josiah Gilbert Holland

Temptation Common to All

Food comes in many forms. What we feed our minds and spirits is just as important as what we feed our bodies. In fact, what we feed our minds and spirits might determine what we feed our bodies. It also might determine what we can resist when it comes to the temptations of physical food.

Jesus knew what it was like to be tempted with food. His answer to that temptation tells us what we should eat.

Matthew 4:1-11 says that Jesus had gone into the wilderness and had fasted 40 days and 40 nights. Naturally, He was physically hungry and weak after such an intense time of prayer and fasting. That was when satan came to Him with an innocent-looking temptation. The devil always tries to trip us at our weakest points.

Jesus had feelings just like ours. He was a man, yet He was God. The Bible says He was tempted in all things, but without sin (Heb. 4:15). His body got tired, hungry, and weak. Still, He was able to face the challenge that satan brought against Him because He was fed with another type of food.

When the tempter came to Jesus, he said, "If Thou be the Son of God, command that these stones be made bread" (Mt. 4:3). The devil tried to raise a question in Jesus' mind about His authority in God. That is one of satan's tactics. He tries to create doubts when we are weak and struggling. He asks questions to cause people to wonder, and then to wander away from God.

The devil tried to deceive Jesus as he had deceived Adam and Eve in the Garden of Eden—asking questions to cause doubt. "If You are the Son of God," he said, "then command these stones to be made bread." Jesus was hungry. He hadn't eaten for 40 days. He was in the wilderness and all about Him were only stones. Jesus could have turned every stone to bread and no one would have known.

But He wasn't supposed to do it. Catering to His physical needs would have made Him a slave to them. It would have weakened His effectiveness and hampered His ministry. If Jesus hadn't conquered the temptation at that moment, satan would have used it against Him later.

Jesus did perform miracles with bread in His ministry. He once fed more than 5,000 people with just five loaves of bread. Great crowds of people began to follow Jesus after that. They wanted more bread. How tempting it must have been for Jesus to turn stones to bread then. It would have satisfied the clamoring crowds and gathered Him more and more followers.

But Jesus knew that His authority did not come from bread. It came from God. Jesus had not come to meet merely the physical needs of mankind; He came to meet our spiritual needs. Bread could never become a substitute for the Word of God.

So Jesus answered the tempter with these words: "It is written, Man shall not live by bread alone, but by every word that proceedeth out of the mouth of God" (Mt. 4:4).

It is not a sin to eat physical food. We must feed our bodies in order to be strong and healthy. But Jesus makes the point here that physical food is not all we need. We need food to sustain the inner person as well. God's Word is this food, as well as positive, uplifting healthy words from other good sources. If we don't feed our spirits and souls, then the physical food we feed our bodies becomes too important. Food will always be a point of weakness where the enemy can defeat us.

Too many people use food as a substitute for satisfying the needs of their souls and spirits. Food becomes a reward or a solace. They try to make food satisfy an emotional need, or even a spiritual need. But bread is a poor substitute for the spiritual food we need to bring health and vitality to our minds, hearts, and spirits.

That is why we must seek food for our minds and our spirits with an even greater diligence than we seek food for our physical bodies. Jesus tells us where to begin that search: in the Word of God.

Jeremiah 15:16 says, "Thy words were found, and I did eat them; and Thy word was unto me the joy and rejoicing of mine heart: for I am called by Thy name, O Lord God of hosts." We can exist on physical food, but we can't really live on bread alone. We truly live when we are whole people, growing, learning, and becoming in every area of our lives. We have to "eat" good words wherever we find them.

This doesn't mean only meditating on the Word of God, although that is a good place to start. I believe there are many sources of good words. As long as those words agree with the principles of the Bible (that's the only way they truly can be good), they can benefit and bless us. So we should meditate on positive thought patterns.

"Thy words were found, and I did eat them." This verse provides an image of sitting down to a wonderful, healthy and positive meal. We derive enjoyment and satisfaction from eating. That's why it's such a temptation to overeat or to eat the wrong foods.

If we eat with our minds and spirits as well as with our bodies, however, the temptation physical food represents will not be as great. It's a matter of strengthening our minds all the time. It is when the mind grows weak that we eat more. We lose our will power and give in to temptation.

Remember, the devil tries to get to people when they are at their weakest points. When you feel that you are under attack, you must do what Jesus did when He was tempted. You must turn to the Word of God. At every temptation, Jesus said, "It is written." He had eaten the Word of God and that gave Him the strength to stand up to the temptation.

If we have eaten good words—God's words—then we can stand up to temptation also. We can tell the devil to leave us alone, in the name of Jesus. This resistance works not only with temptations dealing with food, but also with any other temptation that might come against us.

How does temptation come to us? It comes through the mind. Potato chips, pizza, and chocolate ice cream don't literally chase us down the road demanding to be eaten. The image and desire for food, or anything else, comes through the mind. When we feed our minds with good words and images, then we won't have to feed our minds with thoughts of potato chips, pizza, and chocolate ice cream.

The Power of Words

Can words really make much of a difference in our lives? Does it matter what we put into our minds or our spirits? Yes, words definitely make a difference. You've heard the expression, "The pen is mightier than the sword," and it is true. Words have power—the power of life and death.

Proverbs 4:20-22 says, "My son, attend to my words; incline thine ear unto my sayings. Let them not depart from thine eyes; keep them in the midst of thine heart. For they are life unto those that find them, and health to all their flesh." Good words—words full of wisdom and hope—have life and health in them. They have a power to make a difference in our lives.

Thus, the words you choose to eat will have a powerful effect upon every aspect of your life. They will affect the way you think, the way you behave, and the way you live. They will even affect the food you eat in one way or another.

If you are feeding yourself words of defeat and despair, those words will have a negative effect upon your body, your mind, and your spirit. If you are feeding yourself words of encouragement and hope, then those words will create life and health for every part of your being. Words do make a great difference.

Let's consider some specific words and the power they have. Look at the word *fat*. Does it have the power to evoke an image, to create a feeling, to make us cringe? What about the word *thin*? Its imagery is entirely different; the emotional response it brings may be one of desire or perhaps guilt. Two very small words can create turmoil within us. They have power, and that power does affect our lives.

When you and I put positive words in our hearts, we are putting power and strength in our hearts and spirits. We are building our own faith, our courage, and our will-power. Those words become the ammunition we need to fight discouragement and temptation.

What words you find to consume and meditate upon will either put you under or put you over. They will either defeat you or give you victory. Finding the right words and experiencing the power behind those words may mean the difference between a successful life and a mediocre life.

Eat the Right Words

Here in America, we live in a media-saturated culture. Words bombard us from every side. Television, radio, billboards, bumper stickers, and everything in between carry messages into our brains until sometimes we feel numb to it all. Most of the time we don't think we are even paying attention, but the messages get past the eyes and ears and burrow deep into our subconscious minds.

We've become very health conscious about the foods we eat, carefully watching our sodium and cholesterol intake. But we are usually very careless about our word intake. Some of what we are absorbing into our minds is pure poison.

If we wish to be whole, healthy people, we must watch the words we eat. We must be much more aware of what we are taking into our systems. The words we eat are the words we think on and as we said in the first chapter, what we think is what we become.

Proverbs 16:24 says, "Pleasant words are as an honeycomb, sweet to the soul, and health to the bones." If that principle is true, then the opposite is true as well. Critical, negative words are poison to the soul and destructive to your health. If you struggle with a weight problem or any kind of addiction, you may be hampering your ability to overcome it by eating words that are more destructive than the food you are eating.

I have a friend who was dieting to lose 30 pounds. Someone told him that the first 10 pounds would be easy to lose, but that the last 20 would be hard. Sure enough, he lost 10 pounds quickly and easily. Then he reached a plateau at that weight and could not seem to get any further.

I told him, "You ate those words that you would have a hard time with the last 20 pounds. I think you are subconsciously telling your body to hang on to those pounds and not give them up without a long hard fight. Those words are causing you more trouble than the food is."

He was still eating a healthy, low-calorie diet. There was no physical reason why the eleventh pound couldn't come off just as easily as the tenth pound. His was a mental block with a physical result. He had eaten the wrong words.

He began to tell himself that he could lose those last 20 pounds. He fed himself words of encouragement and faith just as carefully as he fed himself fiber and vitamins, and the weight came off.

There can be all sorts of negative words that hinder us. We may be eating a steady diet of criticism from family, from friends, and even from ourselves. We may be absorbing doubts, fears, rejection, loneliness, and discouragement. All these emotions come with words—words that reinforce the emotions and make them very difficult to overcome.

Perhaps you have been bombarded with the Madison Avenue hard sell that says only tall, thin, blond, tanned people can be happy, successful, rich, and loved. They are the ones who drive the best cars, own the nicest homes, marry the sexiest people, and buy the nicest clothes. You can't hope to measure up, so you feel guilty, unworthy, and unloved.

The words in these commercials might be bright, pretty, happy words; nevertheless, the effect is negative because the message that underlies them is negative. These are words you shouldn't eat. Recognize them for what they are: a way to sell a product. Don't take them into your personal self-image. Don't eat them.

What we want to feed our minds and spirits are positive words, uplifting words, encouraging words, reality words. Remember, Jeremiah 15:16 said, "Thy words were found, and I did eat them; and Thy word was unto me the joy and rejoicing of mine heart...." The right words bring joy and rejoicing. They give us the strength and power we need for healthy living.

The Bible is by far the best source for words of life. Many other good sources also exist, however. Even television, as dubious as that may sound, can offer us good words. Television has been described as "junk food for the mind," but it does offer some good through cultural and educational programing.

We simply must be careful in our choice of the words from the media that we eat. Many times it is a matter of individual make-up. What is poison to one person may be perfectly harmless to another. Educate yourself about what effect words have on you.

The words that give you victory over life and its problems are words that you need to be eating. They don't all have to be Scripture. They don't all have to be deep and profound. Some words might be funny or silly, but if they create a good feeling and a good image, then they are of benefit to you.

Clip cartoons that give you a good laugh. Solomon said that a good laugh was good medicine (Prov. 17:22). Copy uplifting Scriptures that have a strong meaning to you personally. Start a notebook with articles you have read that encouraged you or gave you good information on how to overcome a certain problem. Have a library of good books, tapes, and videos. Then when you get the "munchies," you can eat some good words instead of "junk food."

Here are just a few quotes and Scriptures to get you started in stocking your life with good words to eat. Copy them and keep them handy, or post them around your house where you can snack on them every day.

- I can do all things through Christ which strengtheneth me. (Philippians 4:13)

- Ye are of God, little children, and have overcome them: because greater is He that is in you, than he that is in the world. (1 John 4:4)
- He that sees the invisible can do the impossible.
- You can, if you think you can.
- Nay, in all these things we are more than conquerors through Him that loved us. (Romans 8:37)
- Choice, not chance, determines destiny.
- Finally, brethren, whatsoever things are true, whatsoever things are honest, whatsoever things are just, whatsoever things are pure, whatsoever things are lovely, whatsoever things are of good report...think on these things. (Philippians 4:8)

Eat the Right Images

Just as important as eating the right words is the need to eat the right images. Our minds can create pictures from words. Those pictures, or images, can have just as powerful an effect upon us as the words do. Pictures can play a vital role in what we become because their influence is so great.

In a camera commercial, a tennis star proclaims that "image is everything." In the world of sports and entertainment, that is often true. Stars work very hard at creating an image, one that will focus attention upon themselves. They know that images can have a powerful influence. However, that influence can be either positive or negative.

We must guard our minds from certain images just as we do with words. Sitting in front of the television is too easy sometimes. We don't pay enough attention to what we are watching. We may find ourselves (and especially our children) saying things like, "Hey, dude," and then wondering where it came from.

Do we want to become like Roseanne or the Simpsons? No? Then why do we watch them? Unless we are carefully analyzing what we are hearing and seeing, we may be absorbing these words and images without any protective screening process. You know what they say: garbage in, garbage out.

What about all those food commercials—the ones where everyone who is eating looks healthy, fit, and trim? Anyone who is having trouble with their willpower should examine these commercial images that are steadily bombarding their minds. We might not have a problem with eating food if it weren't for eating the wrong images.

We need to feed ourselves thoughts of discipline, of strength, and of the healthy, fit person we want to be. That means watching what our image intake is. Too many rich, gooey, glamorous, clamorous, lecherous image calories can be bad for one's mental health. Only people bent on self-destruction eat a steady diet of chocolate or french fries. A steady diet of negative images can be just as harmful.

A friend of mine worked for a company where the chairman was a very large man. He weighed more than 300 pounds. We were discussing this book and my friend said to me, "You know, you're right about images. The people who work closely with this man all admire him and respect him and want to be like him. And they are all overweight!"

These people had absorbed the image of a successful, likeable, but overweight, man. They had become what they had looked at day after day.

Whatever we look at all the time—that is what we will become. Those images are going into our minds, into our spirits, into our thinking patterns, into our actions and our abilities. But we are not helpless victims of the images we eat. We can control what we take into our minds. We can put the power of images to work for us by choosing images that build us up and give us strength.

What is your self-image right now? If you described yourself over the phone to someone who had never seen you, what would you say? Would your words be negative? Would you bring up all your faults? Or would you have a few kind words to say about yourself? The way you see yourself comes from the words you have eaten, the thoughts you have entertained, and the images you have taken into your mind.

Image Goals

If your self-image is a negative one, even in part, then you have some work to do. You have some changes to make.

I have a friend, one of the mightiest intercessors for the ministry, who was very overweight. She told me she had this image in her spirit and mind of being like a monster, eating all the time. That was how she saw herself and she had become that very thing. As you can imagine, she was very unhappy and didn't like herself at all. She needed a change of image.

My friend started coming to some of my meetings and God delivered her of that negative vision. She began to see herself as healthy, trim, and self-controlled. She started seeing herself in a new, positive light. Slowly she got her weight under control—because at last she believed she could.

You will always think or meditate on some type of image. I've prayed for people and counseled with them on this matter. Most people who struggle with their weight see themselves as eating, eating, eating all the time. That's the image they have—and that's what must change before they will ever gain control over their eating.

The Bible says, "Keep thy heart with all diligence; for out of it are the issues of life" (Prov. 4:23). You need to keep your image of yourself as pure, clear, and positive as you can. How you see yourself on the inside will be projected on the outside.

God sees you and me in a positive light. To Him we are very beautiful and very special. If you have a hard time believing that, it's probably because you don't see yourself that way. The images you have eaten, perhaps from the time you were a child, have left you with a very different feeling about yourself. But you *can* see yourself in a different light. You *can* see yourself healthy, strong, and whole. All you need to do is reprogram the images in your mind and spirit.

If you have honestly evaluated the image you have of yourself and aren't satisfied with it, then it's time to decide what image you do want to have. What do you want to become?

Do this little exercise. Get a piece of paper and write down a list of words that you would like to describe you. Choose words that would describe every aspect of you—physical, mental, emotional, social, and spiritual. Don't concentrate on only one part of you to the exclusion of all the others. You want to be a whole person.

Be realistic, though. If you are 5′2″, you will not become 5′7″ no matter how many times you write it down or how many images of 5′7″ people you put in your mind. What you need to write down is, "I will be happy being 5′2″." This is a realistic, attainable goal.

Let's suppose someone's list of image goals have these words on it: athletic, beautiful, calm, daring, energetic, fun, gracious, healthy. This person will now want to create images in her mind of being each of these projections. It may take work. It may take overruling some negative images that contradict these goals. But she must daily eat the image of the person she wants to be.

Another way to get good images inside you is to cut out pictures that illustrate what you want to be. If you want to be athletic, cut out a picture of an athlete, preferably one involved in a sport you enjoy. Or find a picture of someone who fits your idea of beauty (everyone sees beauty differently, you know).

Your pictures don't always have to be of people. To illustrate the image of calmness, you might use a picture of a sunset reflected on a quiet lake. Daring could be seen in a mountain climber scaling the heights. Energetic could be portrayed in a child playing with a puppy.

If you were to look at these things every day, don't you think it would have a positive impact on your life? You would be eating the right images—the healthy, positive, vital, victorious images that can help create a new you.

Remember, you are not trying to become the person in these pictures. You are trying to capture the quality that the picture represents. It isn't healthy to try to become another person. It is healthy to become the best you you can be.

Eat the images you want to become. You might keep another notebook for your collection of positive images. You might put up pictures of what you want to become on your mirror or on the refrigerator.

It's all a matter of eating those new images of yourself. After all, you need to gain a new strength if you want to gain a new you. In order to gain that new strength, you must come into new surroundings. You have to surround yourself with pictures of what you want to be like.

Say the Right Words

"I'm fat," Elaine said as she stared into the bathroom mirror. These were the words with which she had greeted herself each morning for the past several months. The forlorn image looking back at her sadly agreed it was true. She had told herself she was fat and her body had complied.

The words she had said to herself weren't always, "I'm fat." At first she said, "No one cares about me." Later she told herself, "I'm worthless." Then it became, "I don't care about myself." Finally it was, "I'm fat." The words eventually became true.

It all began when her husband of 14 years announced that he wanted a divorce. The shock had numbed Elaine at first, but when the final papers were signed, she plunged into a depression that sent her seeking solace from food.

Now she stood in front of the mirror facing a dismal fact. She had become what she had said.

Elaine's story points out one final problem that words and images can create for us. We not only become what we think, and eat, but we also become what we say.

The words that you speak reflect and reinforce whatever images are in your mind. Whatever words and images you have eaten will be the words and images you speak. If it's garbage in, then it's garbage out. If it's health and life taken in, then it will be health and life that comes out.

Proverbs 12:18b says, "...the tongue of the wise is health." It isn't wise to destroy with negative, self-critical words, all the work you did in creating new images in your mind. Wise people will speak healthy words—words that are positive and full of faith. If you are trying to change the way you think, work also at changing the way you talk. Thoughts, words, and actions must all be in agreement if they are to be effective.

Have you ever heard someone (perhaps yourself) say, "If I just look at a piece of cake, I gain five pounds"? Everyone knows that isn't literally true. We don't take in calories through our eyes—thank goodness! It seems like a harmless statement.

But if you do say that, you are actually saying that you gain weight very easily. One piece of cake will put on the pounds. You have an image of yourself gaining weight and you are reinforcing it with your words. Sure enough, you gain the pounds because you look at that piece of cake, make that remark, and eat them both.

It doesn't matter who else hears you make such remarks. You hear you. You have to listen to you talk even if no one else does. So let only positive words, constructive words, healthy words, come out of your mouth. Then you will be hearing and eating the words that bring you victory.

The power of words can never be underestimated. In fact, Proverbs 18:21 tells us, "Death and life are in the power of the tongue: and they that love it shall eat the fruit thereof." The words you speak and the words you eat reveal what you think and what you will become.

What you eat is what you are. Everything you take into yourself in a physical, mental, or spiritual sense, will become who you are. So make wise choices for a healthy life.

Emotional

Chapter 3

Causes and Conflicts

He that respects himself is safe from others; He wears a coat of mail that none can pierce.

—Henry Wadsworth Longfellow

Closely related to the mental aspect of dieting is the emotional aspect. Our emotions are a very important part of our make-up. They greatly influence the way we think, the way we talk, and the way we behave. We cannot change for the better unless we change our emotions as well.

The problem with emotions is their tendency to become tangled and confused. They can also be strong—sometimes stronger than our own will or self-control. Or they can leave us feeling weak and helpless. Very little else in our lives is so dramatic or forceful as our emotions.

It is not surprising, therefore, that negative emotions would have a drastic effect upon the way we live. Likewise, positive emotions can be the force that pulls us up to our very highest level and helps us make the best of ourselves. That is why we must work to keep our emotions healthy and positive, just as we do for our thoughts. The heart is just as important as the mind in living a victorious life.

Our Greatest Need

Have you ever noticed that there seems to be a strong connection between emotions and food? Perhaps it stems from infancy; as babies our greatest needs are to be loved and fed. If we have those two things we are content, we are happy. Things don't seem to change much when we become adults.

Darla's experience is a good example of this. She was engaged to be married after a courtship of three years. Then her fiancé told her that he wasn't ready to get married. Just like that he was gone from her life. I'm sure you can guess what Darla's reaction was. She was hurt and felt rejected and worthless. Her self-esteem plummeted. So she began to eat. It was a way of pampering and consoling herself. Never denying herself anything she wanted to eat was the only way she could feel loved.

Of course, her self-esteem was not helped by the added weight—it only made matters worse. All Darla wanted was to be loved. Unfortunately, she equated love with food and ended up hurting herself even more.

Because Darla worked as a flight attendant, the weight gain was a threat to her job as well as to her health. She knew she had to get things under control so she checked into a health clinic that specialized in eating disorders and weight problems.

The clinic director first gave Darla an emotional profile questionnaire to fill out. By answering those questions, Darla came to understand what food had become to her. It was an emotional substitute. She didn't love herself when she ate. She was actually hurting herself and she learned that it was a deliberate, destructive act on a deep, subconscious level. She was punishing herself by becoming fat because she had no love for herself.

Darla had to change the way she felt about herself. She had to change her thinking and her beliefs. She needed to learn to love herself once again.

We never outgrow the need to be loved. It is a need that we spend our lives trying to satisfy, sometimes even in destructive ways. We want to be loved and admired. We want to be wanted and needed. But can we ever accept love from other people or from God until we love ourselves?

It isn't difficult for babies to receive love. They drink it in as eagerly as they drink a bottle of warm milk. They accept all the care and attention they receive as if it were their due for just being. But that attitude usually doesn't last very long. Sooner or later we all realize that love isn't always given unconditionally. The first bruises inflicted on tiny feelings begin a lifetime of dealing with emotional hurts. Unfortunately, we often develop a low self-esteem from those hurts. We find it hard to love ourselves, and then sometimes we find it difficult to receive love from others.

Our greatest emotional need, then, is for love—not just from God or from the people who are important to us, but also from ourselves. If we don't love ourselves, we won't treat ourselves right. We won't take care of ourselves as we should.

Some people hear the term *self-love* and they think it sounds selfish. After all, as Christians, we are taught to deny ourselves and esteem others as higher. That is all true, but God also said, "Love thy neighbour as thyself" (Lev. 19:18). How can we love our neighbor if we don't love ourselves first?

The value of a healthy self-esteem cannot be overestimated. To feel good about yourself does not mean you are conceited or vain; it means you have understood that because you are God's handiwork, you are of value. God valued you enough to send His Son to die for your salvation. So if you are going around putting yourself down or hating yourself, you are contradicting God. He believes in you. He loves you. Now you too must learn to love yourself.

Loving ourselves does not mean taking on the "me first" attitude that is so prevalent in today's secular society. It doesn't mean that we only "look out for number one." There is a great difference between loving ourselves and being so absorbed with ourselves that we have no time for anyone else. All of us need people in our lives. If we love ourselves, we won't shut others out by being selfish and self-centered.

Yes, love is one of our greatest needs. With love, we can do just about anything. We feel as if we could conquer the world. With love, we are more than a match for anything that comes against us. With love, we are victors, not victims, in this life.

But if love is so important to us, why do so many of us struggle with loving ourselves? There are many reasons.

Obstacles to Love

A well-known minister has said that the extra weight he once carried was like much excess baggage. It didn't belong to him and it only got in his way. Many people carry the excess baggage of emotional hurts inside them, like a great weight that hinders their total health. They struggle with a low self-esteem because of the weights of rejection, criticism, insecurity, disappointment, guilt, and fear.

So many people carry these burdens and cares. Perhaps you are one of them. What emotional "baggage" weighs you down and keeps you from dealing with life in a healthy, productive way? Do you also struggle with a low self-esteem—a lack of love for yourself?

Looking at our emotions can sometimes be harder than examining our thoughts. Emotions are difficult to sort out. They can be deceiving. We may think we are taking care of ourselves, as Darla did, only to find that we have been hurting ourselves.

If we are to be healthy in our emotions, we must look at them honestly. Since almost everyone struggles with emotional hurts, it is safe to say that all of us need to measure our emotions and gauge their impact upon our lives.

Sometimes examining our emotions can be painful. No one wants to relive a moment of rejection, disappointment, or fear. But if you can face these moments in your life and deal with the emotions they caused, you are one step closer to being healthy and whole.

Everyone's "emotional profile" will be different, just as fingerprints are different. You see, you are the sum total of your past experiences. No one else has gone through exactly the same things you have, so they won't feel about things the same way you do.

But there are certain common problems that we all face in one form or another. It is these that damage our self-esteem. They are the obstacles to love that we must overcome.

Rejection

Who hasn't felt rejected at some point in his or her life? It may be as simple as not being chosen for a neighborhood softball team. Or it might be as traumatic as learning your spouse has chosen to divorce you to marry another. The pain may vary in degree, but it is always real.

Darla felt rejected when her fiancé walked out of her life without looking back. It took a long time of discussion in the support group sessions at the health clinic for her to realize that the anger she felt wasn't totally aimed at her financé. Some of it was aimed at herself. Not eating right or taking care of herself was her way of punishing herself because she believed she was unworthy of love.

Darla had to forgive both her former fiancé and herself. Then she had to work on developing self-acceptance. That is something we all need to do.

You will not always be the center of attention. You will not always be the one chosen for that promotion, that role in a play, or that office in a club. That doesn't mean you aren't worthy; it only means you weren't chosen. The fault may not be yours. It may lie with the other person.

You must learn to accept yourself and feel good about yourself. Feelings of unworthiness often cause excessive or unhealthy eating. Whenever you have trouble accepting something about yourself, remember that you are accepted by the two most important people in your life: God and you. The Bible says, "...He hath made us accepted in the beloved" (Eph. 1:6). So don't let people put you under rejection; accept yourself as God does.

Disappointments

Proverbs 13:12 says, "Hope deferred maketh the heart sick: but when the desire cometh, it is a tree of life." How true this verse is. When you hope for something and it doesn't come, it can be very disheartening. That disappointment can then bring pain and bitterness and damage your self-esteem.

In the discussion group at the health clinic Darla was attending, the clinic director told the group how she had overcome disappointment in her own life.

Shelby's dream was to be a doctor. She had completed her undergraduate work in pre-med, but was disappointed time and again when her applications to medical schools were returned.

Shelby did what so many people do when they are disappointed. She ate. By the time she realized what her disappointment was doing to her, she had gained more than 100 extra, unnecessary pounds. The fight back to a healthy weight lasted until she had earned her doctorate in psychology. Shelby then decided to put what she had learned to good use by helping others who struggled with weight problems.

The key to overcoming disappointment is to learn from it. Perhaps that means looking for the proverbial silver lining when gray clouds hide the sunshine in your life.

We all face disappointments. Rains come and cancel planned picnics; relationships fail to bring the fulfillment we desired; circumstances change the direction we wanted to take in our lives. Will you overcome the disappointment or will the disappointment overcome you? If you allow disappointment, lost dreams, or shattered hopes to make you angry or bitter, they will overcome you. Disillusionment can easily lead to a low self-esteem and the self-destructive behavior that accompanies it.

You *can* overcome disappointment. Maybe you will have to change your plans and find new dreams, but you can do it. Disappointments do not have to defeat you. Turn discouraging circumstances into challenging opportunities. Don't let discouragements of the past keep you from enjoying victories today.

Criticism

Critical remarks can create wounds that are slow to heal. When we were children we used to say, "Sticks and stones may break my bones, but words can never hurt me." We said it defiantly, but it wasn't always true. Words can cut deep to our hearts, leaving us uncertain of our worth as an individual.

In the health clinic's support group sessions, 18-year-old Tiffany didn't seem to belong. She was slender, blond, and very pretty. But she told the group that she was anorexic. All her life she had tried to please her critical father, but never succeeded. Nothing she did was satisfactory. She was starving herself because she was starved for his approval and love.

Tiffany had attempted suicide shortly before coming to the clinic. The hospital emergency room had pumped her stomach of the sleeping pills she had taken. When her father finally came to visit her in the hospital, his first words to here were, "Can't you do anything but cause trouble? You're going to pay for this hospital bill! Do you hear me? You'll have to get a job."

Yes, words can be very cruel and leave deep wounds. Few of us have escaped the hurt that comes from criticism. We need to learn, as Tiffany did, that we can never satisfy dissatisfied people. We simply must set our own goals and standards and strive to meet them.

Some people feel that they cannot live up to the standards God has set. These people are fearful of sinning one time too many and falling under His wrath. For them, God is a harsh judge rather than a merciful provider of grace, peace, and righteousness. It is true we will never be as perfect as God, but we can be righteous (which means having a right standing). Jesus offers us His own righteousness.

We can feel good about who we are in Him. We can be pleasing to God and to ourselves. Our worth does not depend upon pleasing anyone else. Now there's nothing wrong with trying to do nice things for the people we love and bringing happiness to them. But our own value as a person does not rest in the words—either good or bad—of someone else.

Insecurity

We've probably all sat in front of the television or flipped through a magazine and sighed at the sight of the beautiful people portrayed there. Even the most attractive people can feel insecure if they are comparing themselves to others. Even those skinny models in the magazines worry about someone more beautiful than they coming along to push them out of the camera's eye.

Insecurities about abilities, intelligence, and appearance plague nearly everyone at one time or another. Anyone who says they haven't worried about a gray hair, an added pound, a report to the boss, or a visit with the in-laws is probably lying. Unfortunately, sometimes we let those insecurities keep us from loving ourselves as we are.

Robert told the clinic support group that he had fought insecurity for most of his life. He had always had a weight problem. Even as a child he was chubby. He could remember chugging around the bases in Little League in a desperate effort to help his team, only to pick himself up from the dust and see his teammates roll their eyes in disgust because he had cost them the game.

"I buried myself in my school books," Robert said, "and consoled myself with more food." He excelled in school, won a scholarship to college, and graduated from law school with honors. But even with a successful law practice, Robert was still shy and insecure. His weight fluctuated up and down because his success on the one hand battled against his feelings of inadequacy on the other hand. Things finally changed when he met his future wife, Stacy.

"Stacy loved me for who I was," Robert explained. "With her encouragement, I'm finally facing things and getting them under control."

You should be able to enjoy your own life without comparing it to others'. If you want to find someone who is better than you in something, you probably can, but what would be the point? You are you—special, unique, created by God. Don't live your life feeling that you don't measure up to someone else.

I was eating at my favorite restaurant not too long ago. One of the waitresses with whom I am acquainted was training a new employee. I asked my friend how the new waitress was doing. She said, "Oh, I don't know. Okay, I guess." There was a tone of jealousy in her voice. The new waitress was quite attractive and I think my friend felt threatened.

Women seem to struggle more with jealousy over appearance than men do. Men tend to be jealous of other men's abilities or achievements. However, regardless of the area or the person experiencing it, jealousy isn't healthy.

Feelings of jealousy, envy, or inferiority can destroy a person's self-esteem. Work to keep such emotions out of your life. They are not healthy and often promote destructive behavior. They can steal your happiness and leave you feeling miserably inadequate. You don't need that in your life. Decide what you want to be and then work to become that without comparing yourself to someone else.

Guilt

Guilt is like the so-called silent killers of high cholesterol level and high blood pressure. It usually isn't seen in our outward emotions. Guilt is something we keep buried deep within us. Often we don't even realize we are carrying the extra baggage around. But its silent work in us can create many problems.

Guilt also is like an acid that eats away at a person. If we feel guilty, we are likely to have a very low opinion of ourselves. We blame ourselves for problems and failures that may or may not be our fault. Whether that guilt is a true or a false guilt, it is still something we must deal with.

Tony was dealing with both true guilt and false guilt when he came to the health clinic. Two years earlier he had abandoned his wife and two children just as his father had left him and his mother when he was a child.

"I always thought it was my fault that Dad left us," Tony told the support group. "For years I went around lying to everybody about what a great childhood I'd had because I was ashamed to say my own father had left me. I vowed I would never do such a thing to my children. But when I lost my job because of my drinking, I figured I was worthless and they'd be better off without me. So I left."

Tony's guilt had created a deep self-hatred. He believed the worst about himself. It took several months of counseling to help him reach a point where he could forgive himself and his father, and seek forgiveness from those he had hurt. Only then was he able to begin the fight to overcome the problems of alcoholism and excessive eating.

Most dictionaries provide two definitions of guilt. One is "the act of having done something wrong." The second is "a feeling of self-reproach resulting from a belief that one has done wrong." Thus there are two kinds of guilt: the true guilt of having done something wrong, and the false guilt of believing you've done something wrong when actually you haven't. Just because you feel guilty doesn't mean you are.

If you are harboring guilt, you must look at it honestly and determine if it is a true guilt or a false guilt. If it is true, then you must try to remedy your wrong and seek forgiveness. If it is false, you must forgive yourself and let go of it. There is no greater waste of emotional energy than feeling guilty about something that isn't even your fault. You don't control the actions of others; don't bear their guilt either.

Fear

Everyone feels fear at one time or another. Some fear can even be healthy if it keeps us from doing some foolish or harmful things. Respect for the very real danger of a storm or a fire is just good common sense. However, many people let fear become a consuming and controlling emotion, and that doesn't make sense at all.

"I guess I'm just a worrier by nature," Trina laughed as she spoke to the support group at the clinic. "And when I worry, I eat."

Fear of everything plagued Trina. She was afraid of storms, afraid of snakes, afraid of heights, afraid of losing her husband to someone else, afraid of offending someone, afraid of making mistakes. Dozens of times as she spoke to the group, she would stop and correct herself as if she were afraid to get any detail of her story wrong. Fear and worry seemed to be her closest companions.

But as Shelby, the clinic director, probed a little deeper, Trina came to realize that fear wasn't simply something that controlled her. Her fears were a way of controlling other people. At her least expression of fear, her husband, children, and friends would rush to her side, consoling and commiserating with her.

Trina's fears brought her the attention she craved. She had no confidence in her ability to get attention in any other way—and the fear provided her with an excuse to eat. Consequently, Trina was reluctant to face her fears and let go of those that were truly unfounded and unhealthy.

Fears can leave you feeling helpless, and that damages your self-esteem. Some fears might even arise from a low self-esteem. In either case, they are unhealthy. If you struggle with fear, look at the causes of the fear honestly. You will know if the fear is reasonable or unfounded. What motivates your worries and fears? Do you seek to control others? Is fear an excuse not to try or not to succeed?

If you are genuinely afraid, you can look to God for His protection and provision. He will bring you peace. If your fear arises from some other motive, then you must face it, deal with it, and let it go. Then you can find healing and health for your emotions.

Reason Rules

The list of unhealthy emotions that damage our self-esteem can include more than the ones we've just reviewed. But these are the basic ones most people struggle with. They point out the need we all have for a strong, healthy self-love.

Are you carrying excess baggage, not realizing the baggage handler is standing by to carry it for you? The Bible tells you to cast your cares upon the Lord (1 Pet. 5:7) and He will carry them for you. With God's help you can gain the victory over the emotions that would threaten you. Don't let those emotions drive you to the refrigerator. Let them drive you to prayer and to action. Build yourself up in confidence and faith.

The negative aspects of life have a way of tearing people down. God builds us up and we too must build ourselves up. We should try to build up one another as well. So free yourself from the condemnation of the past. Refuse to entertain fear, worry, or doubt. Don't harbor rejection, insecurity, or despair.

Cast your cares upon the Lord. Leave them in your place of prayer. Go out with the peace of the Lord. Go out with a song in your heart and a smile on your face. Don't let anybody or anything take your self-love.

It all comes down to deciding whether or not you will be ruled by your emotions or by a reasoned, thoughtful response to life. How do you react to what life hands you? Do you recoil with fear, guilt, disappointment, or insecurity? Do negative emotions color your thoughts dark and dismal? Or do positive emotions make your world bright and beautiful? The choice is yours. Do you control your emotions or do your emotions control you?

Breaking the Patterns

Sometimes you just have to get sick and tired of being sick and tired. It's an old cliché, but it's still true. Only until you are ready to change the patterns of your emotional responses will you be able to overcome those negative emotions.

If you react to every setback and disappointment that you encounter by getting depressed, having a little pity party, and starting to eat, you will want to change that pattern. If every failure or mistake leaves you with self-doubt, insecurity, and fear, you will want to change that pattern. If every "no" you receive makes you feel rejected and unloved and sends you to the refrigerator, then you will want to change that pattern.

We are all creatures of habit. So the responses we make to emotional challenges aren't always carefully thought out. Oftentimes they are just habitual reactions. Something negative happens and we sit down and have a good cry, or mope around the house for a week, or tell everyone who will listen how bad things have been for us. If we thought about what we were doing, we probably wouldn't do it.

It's time to stop and think about your emotions. Take control of how you react. Don't allow anyone or anything to make you angry, sad, or bitter. If you feel any of these things, it is because you have chosen to feel them. You can just as easily choose not to be angry, sad, or bitter. You can choose to be calm, happy, and excited about living. It's time you took control.

Chapter 4

Confidence and Control

It is necessary to the happiness of a man that he be mentally faithful to himself.

—Thomas Paine

Loving Yourself

What would it take for you to feel good about yourself? If nothing short of perfection will do, then you will always be disappointed. But if you set some reasonable goals for yourself, you can learn to like you—even love you—and you can be happy with yourself.

We said earlier that one of our greatest needs is to be loved, yet we are the ones who often deny love to ourselves. Haven't you found that when you make a mistake, you are sometimes harder on yourself about it than anyone else? You worry and fret about it and let it eat away at you for days and perhaps weeks. That isn't healthy. But we all do it at times. We haven't learned to love ourselves.

Most people need to develop a new self-love, a new self-worth, even a new self-image. Remember, the images you feed to yourself are vitally important to what you think and how you act. So a positive self-image will fuel good feelings about yourself and you will be able to love you. The key to developing this new self-image is to decide that you are dissatisfied with the old one. Then you'll be ready to begin again with something better.

After all, you spend more time with you than anyone. If you're not happy with you, that will be reflected in your choices, attitudes, and actions. It will certainly be reflected in your feelings about yourself, and probably in your view of everything around you. A low self-esteem, and in some cases a self-hatred, casts a shadow over your life.

So how do you step into the sunshine and learn to love yourself? Actually, the question should be: How do you re-learn to love yourself? You probably had no problem loving yourself when you were very young. Babies are born with a healthy self-esteem. The hurts that come later are what steal this natural, normal love babies have for themselves.

As adults we sometimes have to work very hard to return to this healthy self-love. It is more difficult for some than for others, depending upon the kind of experiences they had in life. People who faced abuse and neglect have much to overcome. Despite everything, though, we can reach a place where we are able to love ourselves again. We can let the wounds heal and stop living in the past. What happened yesterday is beyond our control. We need to work on successful, healthy living and loving today.

To learn to love ourselves and to develop a healthy life style involves three steps. First, we must make good choices. Second, we must maintain healthy attitudes. Third, we must exercise the proper control.

Good Choices

Someone once said, "We cannot direct the wind, but we can adjust the sails." In other words, we cannot control either circumstances or people; we can only control how we will react to them. The choice is always up to us.

Recently I watched a television talk show that dealt with dieting. One woman on the program had lost and then gained weight in a continuous cycle until she finally looked beyond the food she was eating to why she was eating. She found the root of the problem to be her low self-esteem, brought about by feelings of rejection and insecurity.

Whenever she was hurt or upset, she reacted by eating. So she didn't see her weight gain as being her fault. In fact, everyone told her it wasn't her fault. She blamed situations, circumstances, and feelings.

Finally she realized that she herself chose how she would react to situations and circumstances. She chose how she would feel about what happened to her. At that point she began to make better choices. She lost the weight and was able to maintain the loss without gaining it back. She said she would never again give her health to anyone or anything outside of herself.

Most people believe their feelings are beyond their control. "I can't help how I feel," they say. We have this idea that emotions jump on us from the outside. Love comes when Cupid hits the mark with his arrow. Anger comes when someone or something "makes" us angry. Self-pity or sorrow comes because of circumstances or actions of others.

The truth is, emotions rise from within us. If we feel love, anger, self-pity, or sorrow, it is because we choose to feel these emotions at a deep inner level. That level is so deep we may not even realize that we are making such a choice. We think these feelings come unbidden and uncontrolled.

Many times we react to certain situations out of habit. We always reacted this way, so we think we always will react the same. There seems to be no choice. Since these reactions are automatic, we usually don't exercise a conscious choice about them. But if we are not satisfied with those reactions, we then have the power to change them. It's just a matter of *choosing* to change them.

Since habits can be hard to break, it may take work to change those automatic reactions. If certain situations always make you angry, it may take time to change that reaction. Just because you decided to change does not mean you'll suddenly be in control of your anger. It may take weeks of practice to form a new habit, or a new reaction. Making the choice not to be angry is something you must do over and over again until it becomes your new habit.

Once you begin to make choices and changes about how you feel, changes in your behavior will likely follow. If disappointment always made you feel sorry for yourself, which in turn made you head for the kitchen, a new choice in how you feel can change what you do.

The point is to make you realize that your feelings are not at the mercy of outward circumstances. No one has the power to make you angry or sad. People may do things that deserve anger or sorrow, but they cannot force those emotions upon you.

Whether or not you love yourself depends upon whether or not you *choose* to love yourself. It doesn't depend upon whether someone else loves you, what you look like, or what you have done in your life.

Chances are that you are not a perfect person anyway. Who is? Perfection isn't what matters. What does matter is how you see yourself—how you feel about yourself. Is it good or bad?

There may be many things you don't like about yourself. Everyone could probably say that about themselves. But you will never become any better than you are now until you decide that you are worth the effort it will take to change. When you decide that you love yourself enough to better yourself, you've made a choice that can change your entire life.

It's a wonderful thing to be able to say, "I love myself enough to not overeat or fill my body with junk." There is power in being able to say, "I love myself enough not to let other people control how I feel." There is freedom in saying, "I love myself enough not to be bound by bad habits, negative thoughts, or destructive emotions."

Choose to Be the Best You

What is best for you may not be best for someone else. Loving yourself may mean going against the crowd in some ways. It may mean having to tell your mother you don't want a second helping of her meatloaf. No one said this would be easy.

When you begin to make choices for yourself that are based upon loving yourself and wanting to take care of yourself, you may expect some opposition from those who want you to stay the way you are. People who want to be successful may be viewed by others as a threat. If you change, you will upset the status quo—and that may upset some people in your life. This is the dilemma that often makes change so difficult.

Feeling good about yourself doesn't mean you ignore the feelings of others. If the people who are closest to you appear uneasy about the changes you are trying to make, you may have to discuss the situation with them honestly. I believe that anyone who truly loves you will understand your desire to improve.

Once they understand that any changes you make in yourself will not threaten your relationship with them, they will probably become your biggest cheerleaders. That can be so important when you are fighting old, stubborn habits and thoughts.

But remember, you look at yourself more than anyone else does. You listen to you more than anyone else does. You bear the consequences of your decisions and actions more than anyone else does. Only God knows you better than you do. Only you and God can decide what choices you need to make to be your best. You must follow what God is speaking to you in your heart. If choices are from God, they will not only be good for you, they will be good for others. So don't be talked out of becoming a better you.

Tiffany, the pretty 18-year-old mentioned in Chapter 3, received no support from her family when she began to overcome her low self-esteem and the resulting anorexia. Her mother fretted because Tiffany was becoming much more independent and strong-minded. "You're changing, Tiffany," she would say. "I don't know you anymore. What are those people at the clinic doing to you?"

Her father simply ridiculed her efforts to change. He was threatened by the new Tiffany because he could no longer control her every thought and action. So he in turn threatened to kick her out of the house. As Tiffany blossomed under the love of the clinic support group, she grew strong enough to make the decision herself to get a job, enroll in the local junior college, and move into an apartment of her own.

Some people will face opposition such as Tiffany did. Fortunately, just as many of us will find support from our family and friends. Of course, we always will find support from God. He will be there for us even if no one else is. The Bible says, "...He which hath begun a good work in you will perform it..." (Phil. 1:6). In other words, what God starts, He finishes. He created each of us and He will see us through to the end.

You can choose to be your best. Being your best doesn't mean being like everyone in your church or like your favorite preacher. Too often we in a church try to get others to conform to our idea of what is right and best. When new people join our church, we expect them to talk, dress, and act like we do.

The Bible certainly sets the same standards of conduct for all of us. God doesn't play favorites. Still there is plenty of room in the Kingdom of God for us all to be ourselves—our best selves. We should love ourselves enough to make this choice.

The important thing to remember is to keep the emotions in balance. Keep your emotions consistent with the love you are developing for yourself. The consistency of good thoughts, good words, good images, and good feelings will determine the consistency of your healthy, happy life.

Do your best to be happy so you won't give in to the wrong voices, the ones that drive you to do what you don't want to do. Remember, your happiness is not based on outward circumstances. You must choose to be happy. How you feel about yourself makes you happy or unhappy. In fact, you can be happy where you are right now; it just depends upon your attitude.

Changing Attitudes

I suppose our feelings or emotions could be called the thoughts of the heart. Therefore, just as we want to keep the thoughts of the mind positive and uplifting, so we want to keep the thoughts of the heart positive and uplifting.

We said that loving ourselves and living our lives in a healthy way depends upon our making right choices and maintaining healthy attitudes. Our attitudes are the thoughts of our hearts. They are a combination of what we feel and what we think.

Let's look more closely at attitudes. Suppose there is a person in your life whom you have a bad attitude toward. You just don't like that person. (We won't judge the rightness or wrongness of that right now. We just want to look at the attitude.) Perhaps that person works in your office or attends your church. Your personalities seem to clash all the time. Probably everyone has experienced this—except, perhaps, for Will Rogers.

Now think about how you react to this person every time you see him. The first thing you get is an unpleasant feeling down inside. This is followed by a negative, critical thought or maybe several negative thoughts. Suddenly your day seems less pleasant. You feel out of sorts and out of control. You have an "attitude."

There may or may not be serious consequences in your life because of this attitude. It depends upon how well you can control it. But suppose the "attitude" you have is toward yourself. If that is the case, you will have a hard time loving yourself and taking care of yourself as you should. The consequences of this bad attitude could be keeping you from being the person you want to be.

Do you get up in the morning, stumble into the bathroom, look in the mirror, and instantly have a negative reaction to you? First comes the feeling, then comes the critical thoughts, and that is usually followed by negative words. Do you say to your reflection, "Boy, you look terrible this morning"?

To say that to anyone else would be rude, yet we routinely say such things to ourselves if we have a bad attitude toward ourselves. That must change if we are to ever overcome a weight problem or any other problem holding us back from being our best. To change the words, thoughts, and feelings, we must change the attitudes of the heart.

If you don't feel good about yourself, it will show in your attitude toward yourself and probably toward the people and circumstances in your life. I've known people who go through life being miserable and making everyone around them miserable simply because of an unhealthy attitude toward life. People who don't like themselves can usually find something wrong with everyone and everything else. Nothing satisfies them because they have such a negative attitude.

Eddie had such an attitude. He went through life acting as though everyone owed him something because he grew up with few economic advantages. Even though he was a gifted athlete, he struggled with a low self-esteem. Like many boys, he thought basketball was his ticket to a better life. For a while it seemed to be true. But while Eddie's bank account changed, his attitude didn't.

Eddie was rude, abrupt, and often moody. People put up with his attitude because he was a valuable asset to the team. But a knee injury meant Eddie would be off the court for a year and would need extensive therapy to get back to playing condition. Eddie wasn't willing to work that hard. He wanted everything handed to him.

He took a managerial position in the team's front office and suddenly no one was willing to overlook his complaints and critical remarks. Eddie found himself with few friends. He started drinking and putting on weight because he quit working out. His wife took all she could stand of him and then left him, taking the children. Eddie was left with just his attitude.

Eddie ended up back in his old neighborhood, back where the crippling negative emotions had first developed. Then one day he walked by the old city park where he used to play ball with the boys. A game was going on just as it had when he was a kid. A kid playing there reminded Eddie of himself when he was that age.

But this kid was different. He played with determination, yet he looked as if he was enjoying himself too. The other kids seemed to like him. He never lost the smile on his face even when he missed an easy shot. Then the kid fell, grabbing his knee. The others gathered around him and it was like an instant replay of Eddie's own injury.

But the kid got up, grinned at the hole in his jeans, and hobbled over to a bench. The others went on with the game, but Eddie watched this kid. He kept flexing his knee, wincing a bit, and before long he was back in the game. Eddie walked away, but that was the day he started working on a whole new attitude.

Negative emotions are like extra, unwanted baggage. Negative attitudes can be too. They can stand in the way of progress in every area of your life. If you are carrying around a bad attitude toward yourself or someone else, you're hurting your chances of succeeding in life. That attitude will have to go.

The other day a friend of mine said to me, "It's easy to see what someone else is going through, but it's hard to figure out things in your own life." I know what she means. Sometimes it's hard to identify the problem areas in our own lives because we are so close to them that we can't see them. So when an attitude is tangled up with a strong emotion, it's even harder to sort things through and find what changes we need to make.

To determine if you are being hampered by negative attitudes, ask yourself a few questions.

- With what emotions, thoughts, and words do I begin my day? Are they consistently positive or negative?
- When bad things happen to me, do I feel that I deserve them? Do I feel sorry for myself? Do I try to get other people to feel sorry for me?
- When someone pays me a compliment, can I accept it graciously or do I put myself down? Can I compliment others and give them credit for a job well done? Do I need all the attention for myself?
- Am I always expecting the worst to happen? Am I surprised when things turn out well? Am I suspicious when people do nice things for me?

I think the answers you give to these questions will help you discover if your attitudes need changing. Hopefully this small list of questions helped spark some ideas of your own about your feelings and the attitudes they created within you. After all, your attitudes can be like your habits. You get so used to them that you are not always aware of them. So you need to recognize the problem before you can do anything about it.

The way to deal with an attitude is to deal with its roots—your feelings and thoughts. It's just like trying to get unwanted dandelions out of your lawn. If you don't get the roots, you'll be looking at them again next spring. Attitudes change when feelings and thoughts change.

You can be rid of the self-pity syndrome. Or do you want people feeling sorry for you all the time? After all, what does that do for you? You get people to pay attention to you, but it's a negative form of attention that only reinforces your negative attitude. When you get rid of the self-pity syndrome, you give people a good reason to pay attention to you.

You can overcome the "I can't" attitude. You don't have to feel overwhelmed all the time. Start believing in yourself and you will be surprised to find that you can do a lot more than you ever knew.

You also can be free of the "I'm worthless" feeling. No one is worthless. You can see value in other people; see value in yourself as well.

You change such negative attitudes as these by replacing them with healthy ones. The mind is not a vacuum, and neither is the heart. Fill both with positive feelings—even if they are not strong ones at first. With time they will grow stronger, and so will you.

Developing Discipline

All this leads to the third step in developing a loving, healthy life style: exercising control in our lives. We must learn to be in charge of our thoughts, our feelings, and our actions. If we surrender control to someone or something else, then we are always at their mercy. We would never accomplish the changes we want to make in our lives.

This matter of control, however, can be a tough one to manage. The eating disorders of anorexia and bulimia are often control gone awry. In urging you to take control of your life, I must also caution you not to let control become an obsession. That's why I say we must exercise the "proper" control.

Eating healthy does not mean starving yourself. There is nothing healthy about that. People who suffer from anorexia and bulimia often feel that they have no control in their lives. The only thing they can control is the food they eat, so they go overboard with that control and it becomes a life-threatening problem. If you suffer from either of these diseases, please seek medical attention. Don't let too much control in this one area kill you.

The control that you exercise in your life should be one of a healthy self-discipline. You know what is good for you and what is bad for you. If you don't, this book and many other good books can help you learn. Once you know the good from the bad, however, it's up to you to discipline yourself. No one else can do it for you. There is no guardian angel who will slap our hands every time we reach for a potato chip. The discipline and control is up to us.

Neither can you look to family and friends to control you. Even if they were willing to do so, after a while you would resent them. You will find yourself slipping around behind their backs. Besides, no one can control the inside things of thoughts and emotions except you.

What about God? Won't He discipline and control us if we surrender to Him? God does want us to surrender our lives to Him. We can't make a better move than that in getting started on a healthy, abundant life. But even God won't force us to be good. He has given us a free will, and He never violates that.

He will speak to us quietly, inside, guiding us in knowing what is right and wrong. But it is still our decision as to whether or not we will listen and obey His voice.

How you think, how you feel, and how you behave are your decisions. Feed yourself good thoughts, images, words, and food, and you will be good. Every day that you exercise discipline and control will help you grow stronger.

We can control neither the circumstances around us nor what people say or do. But we can control what we listen to, what we believe, and what we do. We can control what we eat or don't eat. One woman has said, "If I want to eat, I consider whether it is for a nutritional or an emotional need. It if is for an emotional reason, I take control and direct my attention and focus to something else."

Food is often used as an emotional escape. But so are many other things: television, sleep, shopping, the telephone. Anything that keeps us from dealing with the emotions and thoughts of the moment are escapes that need to be controlled. Often these things are just thoughtless habits, but if they keep us from facing life squarely, they can hurt us in the long run. We must take control.

Boredom is another excuse for excessive eating. If you have time on your hands, do you reach for food to fill that time? Many people eat, not because they are hungry, but simply because it is something to do. As you develop more interests and activities in your life, the boredom will be replaced with challenge and excitement.

If you are shutting down your life because you don't want to deal with some emotional pain, you are hurting yourself in many ways. You must gain control over the boredom, as well as the frustration and bad habits it creates, by facing life squarely and gaining control over yourself.

I saw a man being interviewed on a talk show. At one time he had weighed 587 pounds. His family and friends told him repeatedly that if he didn't get his eating under control, it would eventually kill him. It almost did. After a severe heart attack, he finally realized that he had to get some control in his life. Over several years, he lost 417 pounds!

This man was a Christian and he realized that God, through His grace, had given him choices for his life—good and bad. Genesis 1:28 tells us that

God gave man authority and dominion over the earth. "How can I control things on earth if I can't control myself?" the man asked. "How can I have the image of Christ in me if I can't control my own life? I'm living a lie." That realization gave him the strength and discipline to change.

He no longer eats a dozen eggs for breakfast and a whole chicken for dinner. He says food no longer excites him. He has found more important things in life through choice, attitude, and control.

Proverbs 16:32b says, "and he that ruleth his spirit [is better] than he that taketh a city." The battle to control yourself is much more difficult to win than a battle over some outside force. If you can develop the discipline it takes to control you, then you have found the key to conquering anything.

Strength and Conviction

As you develop new thoughts and new emotions, you'll find that you can finally get off the dieting merry-go-round. The majority of people who go on a diet and lose weight will eventually gain it all back. That's because reducing calories is only a very small part of maintaining a healthy weight and life style.

I know of a woman who was always on a diet. She could lose weight easily but always gained it back. Finally she had to stop and look at why the diets failed her. She said, "The outside of me changed but the inside didn't. I still had problems with all those old attitudes."

During the time she was dieting, she was going through two consecutive, difficult marriages, both of which ended in divorce. She had let the men in her life put her down because she had a low opinion of herself. Then she began to examine her life and found that she needed to make changes on the inside. "Now I get to work at loving me thin," she says. "Fat may be my size for now, but it is no longer my attitude."

This woman finally found the strength she needed to maintain healthy attitudes and to develop a healthy way of life. A diet is only as good as the healthy thoughts and emotions that accompany it. If you're putting unhealthy thoughts and images into your mind, if you're holding on to negative emotions and attitudes in your heart, then even the most nutritious foods will not have a lasting impact on your body.

Everything worth accomplishing in life requires strength and a conviction to work at it. Strength and conviction come when you have established a healthy state of mind and heart. "I love myself enough that I'm not going to eat junk. I love myself enough that I'm not going to listen to put-downs. I love myself enough that I'm not going to carry around the extra baggage of negative emotions and harmful thoughts."

Getting the strength and conviction is one thing; holding on to it is quite another. Most of us can begin well in making changes, but somewhere down the line we get tired, we let down our guard, and before we know it, we have slipped back into the old patterns. How do we keep the determination alive? How do we make the changes last? How do we keep the control in the proper perspective?

The people who succeed at anything in life are those who decided beforehand to never give up. So here are some tips for keeping strength and conviction working in your own life.

- Know what you want to achieve. Have a strong image, a big goal, and the desire to achieve it.
- Make up your mind that you can succeed. Forget the past and its problems or failures. Nothing has to hold you back.
- Accept the responsibility for your own life. Don't make excuses. Hold yourself accountable for your thoughts, emotions, and actions.
- Determine that you will not quit no matter what happens. Believe in your dream and in your ability to accomplish it.
- Keep your plan before you. Write down your goals in specific detail. Make an image book with pictures and review it often.

- Take one day at a time. Start where you are and work at changing slowly but consistently.
- Say what you want out of life, not what you don't want. Say that you can succeed and you can achieve.
- Surround yourself with supportive people who aren't intimidated by your desire for success.
- Avoid drudgery, boredom, frustration, hopelessness, and other things that hold people back from going in the right direction. Make achieving your goals challenging and fun.

You will have many victories, but you also will have battles. Hold on to what you have gained. Never give back any ground. Keep pressing forward and you will achieve in life what you have determined to do and be.

Physical

Chapter 5

Setting New Goals

One should eat to live, not live to eat.

—Benjamin Franklin

Most diet books begin and end with the physical aspect of dieting, but as we have shown in the previous chapters, our bodies are only one part of who we are. Because the body is the most visible part of us, we often focus most of our attention on it when losing weight.

In fact, in today's culture, we seem almost obsessed with the idea of having the perfect body. All the emphasis we put on beauty and strength center around the body. We so easily forget or ignore the fact that beauty and strength are qualities of the spirit and the soul that are merely reflected in the body. To pay attention to only the physical aspects of life is to limit ourselves. Whole people are more than just beautiful bodies.

That is why the chapters dealing with the physical part of us are tucked in the middle of this book. We can't ignore our bodies in the hope that they will be healthy and fit on their own, but neither should we be so obsessed with them that we can think of nothing else. Balance is the key to dealing with the visible, physical part of us.

Finding the Balance

How important is your body to you? The answer to this question will not be the same for every person. Some people are in professions where a trim, attractive appearance is considered part of the job. For those people, maintaining a certain weight may be very important. For other people, how much they weigh may not concern them at all except in terms of being healthy.

You must decide for yourself how much emphasis you want to place on your body. The point is, don't be pressed into someone else's mold. You don't have to weigh the precise amount as some skinny model or some muscle-bound athlete. Be an individual and find out what is right for you.

It's very easy to find a chart that will tell you what is the most healthy weight for someone of your height and age. Most of these charts will give a range of perhaps five to ten pounds—or even more—that is healthy. There is no ideal weight just as there is no ideal color of hair, skin, or eyes. What is best for each person is an individual matter.

If you have decided that you are not happy with your body as it is right now, then you have the choice to change it. But don't try to change it to fit into someone else's clothes or life style. Change it to fit you. Find your own balance for reaching the place you can feel good about yourself.

I'm sure you've heard the expression, "You can never be too rich or too thin." That is a very revealing statement; it tells us what our society emphasizes the material and the physical.

That expression is false and misleading. I don't know if you can be too rich and I'm not in any danger of finding out! But I do know it is possible to be too thin. You can lose too much weight. Being too thin can be very unhealthy. It can cause enormous health problems, some of which can even be fatal.

The late Karen Carpenter is proof of that. Though she was extremely popular, successful, and probably rich, she was also anorexic. Her obsession with her weight put everything in her life out of balance. Years of unhealthy diets eventually weakened her heart and resulted in her tragic death.

So there is "thin" and there is "too thin." Thin can be very healthy; too thin is not healthy at all. At the same time, there is "fat" (for lack of a better word) and "too fat." Just because someone is a large person does not necessarily mean that person is unhealthy. It is only when an individual becomes "too large" that he endangers his health. The point when a person becomes "too fat" or "too thin" is an individual matter. That point will be different for you than it is for me or for anyone else.

You must find out what is healthy for you by finding your own healthy weight range. It may be a range as wide as 20 or 30 pounds. You may be able to weigh 20 pounds more than someone else of the same height and age and suffer no ill effects from that extra weight. Or you may experience health problems by being only five or ten pounds over the recommended weight. It all depends upon the condition of your own body.

How Much Is Enough?

You know when you feel good and when you don't. If you feel fine, but people are urging you to lose weight, you must decide for yourself if you want to do it. Don't be pressured into dieting just to conform to someone else's idea of what is good for you.

Always check with your physician before taking on the challenge of losing a large amount of weight. If you have just a few pounds to lose, you can probably do it safely and easily without a physician's care. But if it will be a drastic change, be sure to get advice from your doctor.

Your doctor will also be able to tell you if your weight is creating health problems you might be unaware of. As we said, losing weight should be for the sake of health, not conformity to some elusive Hollywood ideal. If you choose to lose weight, do it for yourself—your health and your own self-esteem. Don't do it because of the television commercials or magazine advertisements.

However, you don't want to use nonconformity as an excuse not to reduce your weight if it truly is a health hazard. It's little consolation to say, "I don't have a problem with my weight" if you are in the hospital after suffering a heart attack. You may want to believe you don't have a problem with your weight, but if it's creating havoc with your health, you have a problem.

There are at least three sources that can tell you what is the best weight for you: your own understanding of how your body functions best; your physician's advice; and standardized weight charts. Taking all three into consideration, what is the best weight range for you?

You will notice that I use the phrase "weight range." No one will weigh the exact same amount of pounds throughout their whole lives. Most of us don't even maintain the exact weight all year round.

It probably isn't possible, and it isn't necessary for good health. What you are looking for is a range of weight that you can stay within and still be healthy and happy.

In boxing, there are many different weight divisions: featherweight, lightweight, middleweight, heavyweight, and so on. Each of these weight divisions has a range that the boxer's weight must fall within. A boxer such as Sugar Ray Leonard doesn't weigh the same as one like Evander Holyfield. They pick the division that is best for them to maintain, and then they work within that range.

You can do the same thing. It's perfectly okay to select a specific weight as a goal when you are trying to lose some pounds. But don't get upset if your weight varies a little from that goal from time to time. It doesn't mean you have failed. It only means you are normal. If you put on a few extra pounds during the holidays (most of us do!), then you know you must work those pounds off when you become more active in the spring. It's all a part of the cyclical pattern of nature.

If you have pets, you may have noticed that they tend to eat more in the winter than they do in the summer. My cat seems to eat quite a bit more during cold weather. He needs the extra body weight to insulate him from the cold. When the weather warms, he sheds the pounds along with his heavier winter coat of fur. This is the instinctive wisdom that God has placed within animals.

We human beings could use some of this wisdom. Instead we let fashion and a jumble of emotions and thoughts get in the way of plain common sense. We become easily frustrated and even obsessed with keeping our weight perfect and we make ourselves perfectly miserable in the process.

So the answer to "How much is enough?" is something each individual decides. You choose what weight you want to maintain, within a flexible range. You decide how much you need to lose or to gain. Make this decision based upon the dictates of your own desires and health, not on someone else's standards. Once you've made a wise, healthy choice, then you'll be ready to begin the work.

Setting Goals

Patricia was always on a diet. But she never seemed to get anywhere in her dieting because she never decided where she wanted to go. Her weight goals were vague and always changing. As a result, Patricia was continually frustrated. She went from one diet to another, thinking that if she could find the perfect diet, the pounds would magically fall away. Of course, she never found the perfect diet.

Perhaps you know someone like Patricia, or maybe you see a little bit of yourself in her story. If you are always trying to "lose some weight," but never seem able to do it, you may need to change your goal. Or maybe you need to get a goal.

How much do you want to weigh? How many pounds must you lose to reach that weight? If you plan to lose more than 15 or 20 pounds, it would be a good idea to break your goal into two or three stages.

First, choose a specific date by which you want to reach your weight goal. Don't be vague and say you want to lose weight "someday." Someday seldom ever comes. Pick a date and circle it on the calendar. Take into consideration how much you want to lose and give yourself an ample amount of time to do it. If you set an unrealistic date, you will quickly become discouraged and give up.

Plan on losing about a pound a week. That is a safe and sane rate to take weight off and keep it off. You can lose weight at a faster rate if you choose, but then you run more risks in terms of health and morale.

Of course, if your doctor advises that you need to lose weight more quickly because you are at a health risk if you don't, then follow his advice and supervision. Rapid weight loss should always be regulated by your doctor.

Once you have established your goal of how much you want to lose and when you want to reach your target weight, then you should break it down into stages. Usually three stages of short, medium, and long-term goals are adequate.

Setting goals in three stages serves two purposes. First, it keeps you from getting discouraged if the weight comes off slowly. Second, it lets you know if the rate you have set is a realistic one. If you have trouble reaching your short-term goal, you may decide to adjust the next two goals to a more realistic schedule.

Mark all three of your goals on a calendar with the amount you desire to lose by each date. Keep the calendar out where you can often see it. This is meant to be a motivating factor, not a sword hanging over your head. If you find yourself having trouble reaching your goals, you can re-evaluate those goals. You may have to adjust the goals or adjust the diet. But don't quit! You can reach your ultimate goal if you don't give up.

Remember, you probably didn't gain the extra weight overnight. You won't lose it overnight either, and there is no reason to expect that you will. Sometimes we want to lose weight by a certain date—prom night, wedding day, important job interview, etc. If you start your diet program in plenty of time, you can reach such a goal. But if you don't give yourself enough time, you will end up being frustrated and disappointed. Then you will be tempted to try one of those unhealthy crash diets. Your emotions, instead of reason, will rule you, and chances are you will gain weight instead of losing it.

This is the cycle that so many people follow. It's another reason some people are always on a diet. The goals they set are unrealistic; they become upset and their self-esteem plummets; they eat more instead of less to satisfy the emotional need; and they think they are a failure because the diet didn't work.

Very often the binges that people go on result from unrealistic expectations. They mistakenly think they have failed at the diet, so they throw the whole thing out the window and eat everything in sight. Binges are very closely tied to our emotions and they can further destroy our confidence.

I don't think anyone has gone on an eating binge who hadn't first been on an unsatisfactory diet. But of course, binging only makes the goal harder to reach and leaves us even more frustrated. So we try another diet—and another and another—never realizing that the diet wasn't what failed; it was the unrealistic expectations we had established for ourselves.

So maybe you won't weigh the perfect weight on that important day. Don't let it discourage you from continuing to strive for a healthy weight. You have the rest of your life to live even after a certain day has come and gone. You want the rest of your life to be as healthy and happy as you can make it. Set goals for all of your life; not just as a one-time effort. Decide what you want to be, then do what you have to do.

New Behaviors

Obviously, if you want to change your weight, you must change something else as well. The calories won't burn and the pounds won't melt away just by wishing they would. What you change, though, depends on what you learned needs to be changed as you read this book. It may be the way you think. It may be the images and words you eat. It may be the way you deal with your emotions.

All of these changes may be necessary for a change in your diet to be effective and lasting. As you begin to take more control of your life, make healthy choices, and develop positive attitudes, then you will be ready to take care of the food.

We said at the beginning of this book that dieting has only a little to do with food. Successful dieting has as much to do with the way you think, feel, and act as it does with what you eat. That doesn't mean what you eat isn't important to your health. Food is only one piece of the puzzle, but it is a key piece.

Once you decided you were ready to make some changes and you set some realistic goals, then you are ready to take care of the more mundane, day-to-day chore of changing your relationship with food.

The first step in changing your food intake is to understand how you eat at the present moment. Take some time to study your eating patterns. Do you eat at certain times of the day? Do you eat when certain things happen, or when your emotions are at a certain level? What kinds of food do you eat? What are your weaknesses—junk food, chocolate, pastries, ice cream?

Once you have identified the problem areas in your eating habits, you can begin to change them. Don't expect overnight success in this, either. Habits form over a period of time, and that is how they are broken. By the time you reach your target weight, you should have replaced your bad eating habits with good ones.

Physical Changes

1. Most of us eat at regular time periods. When our noon break comes, we eat lunch whether we are hungry or not. One of the simplest and easiest ways to cut down on our food intake is to eat only when we are truly hungry. So keep active; don't let eating become your pastime. Fill vacant moments of time with hobbies or small tasks that keep you busy and away from the kitchen.

2. The problem with sitting down to a big, delicious meal is we tend to eat more than we need. If you get up from every meal feeling stuffed, you are eating more than your body actually needs to be healthy and active.

If you are the food preparer, perhaps you need to cut back on the amount of food you put on the table. Don't feel that you must have a meat, bread, or potatoes at every meal.

Learn to recognize when you have reached the point of having eaten enough. You will feel satisfied but not uncomfortable. Eat until you are fine, not until you are full.

3. Unless your eating habits are absolutely atrocious, you are probably eating many healthy foods already. Try to increase that amount of healthy foods to 80 percent of your diet. Then when you want to splurge occasionally, you can. If time constraints require a fast-food meal now and then, it won't be devastating because you would have balanced it with plenty of fruits, vegetables, and grains.

4. Many of us make the evening meal our biggest meal of the day largely because that is when we have the most time for food preparation. But the later we eat, the less time we have to digest the food before going to sleep. If the evening meal is your largest meal, eat it as early as you can. If possible, make lunch your large meal, which gives your body plenty of time to process those calories and burn them more efficiently.

Environmental Changes

1. What foods occupy your kitchen cabinets right now? If you don't buy junk food and keep it around

the house, you will be far less likely to eat it! Stock up on healthy snack foods such as fruits and vegetables and low sodium, low fat crackers. If you do buy those tempting foods such as ice cream, chips, or cookies, get them in single serving sizes so the amount you eat at one time is limited.

2. Is the grocery store your favorite place to shop? Here in America, we are blessed to have almost any food readily available to us. But sometimes that blessing can be a problem. If you find yourself filling your shopping cart with too much food or the wrong kinds of food, you may need to change the way you shop.

Try going to the store only once or twice a week. For some reason, we don't like to run into the store for only one or two items. So we find ourselves buying several things that we really don't need. Eliminate those quick stops by careful planning. Be sure to eat before doing your weekly shopping, too. That food is all the more tempting if you are hungry when you shop.

3. Eating ahead of time is also a good idea when attending parties or other functions where food is served. A buffet-type service is particularly tempting. Choose low calorie items such as fresh vegetables or seafood to munch on and drink bottled water or a diet soda. If you plan ahead, you can avoid being caught off guard or with your defenses

down. You won't find yourself in tempting situations as often.

Mental and Emotional Changes

We have already covered these changes in the preceding chapters, but we will review them here briefly. That way you'll have a complete summary you can refer to quickly.

1. Develop thinking patterns that are positive and uplifting. Remember, you are what you think. Dwell on what you can do, not on what you can't do. Avoid thoughts that depress you or discourage you.

2. Once you have developed an understanding of what you believe about yourself, you can work on strengthening positive beliefs. Learn to feel good about yourself even if you aren't perfect—yet. Reinforce your positive thoughts and feelings with positive words.

3. Identify the emotions that may trigger eating. Remember that choice, attitude, and control are within your power. No emotion, circumstance, or individual can make you eat if you choose not to.

4. Establish goals for your life and keep those goals before you. Write them down, tape them, make an image book. Eat good words and positive images until they become a part of you, and you become what you want to be.

5. Develop a support group. Share honestly with family and friends about your goals. Ask for their help. As much as you politely can, avoid the people who would discourage you or who create tension and trigger negative emotions within you.

Now, none of the changes included here are truly difficult to make. Some are quite simple, yet effective. You can reach your weight goal by the target date you have chosen if you think of the changes you make as life style changes, not just as food changes. What you want to become is healthy and whole, not just thin.

Eating Healthy

Do you hate the word *diet*? Marjorie did. She said it was one of the reasons she never had much success in trying to lose weight. "Saying you were on a diet sounded like you were depriving yourself of something," she said. "I developed this martyr complex every time I tried to diet. I ended up feeling sorry for myself and then I would blow the whole diet with an eating binge."

If dieting sounds like hard work, or causes you to feel deprived, or drives you to a pity party after a few days, then perhaps you need to use a different term to describe the process. Remember, the success of your attempts to lose weight depends largely upon what you think and how you feel. If you hear the word "diet" and have a negative reaction to it, that will undermine your efforts and threaten your success.

Use a phrase such as "new eating program." If you include the word *eating,* it won't feel so much like you're depriving yourself of something you enjoy. You won't stop eating; you simply will eat differently. You approach the matter of food with different thoughts, feelings, and actions.

In a sense, you eat your way to good health. Unless your doctor has put you on a very strict diet, you won't drastically reduce your calorie intake. You just change it. You continue eating, but the foods are different—they're better for you. Your attitude toward food changes; it no longer is so important to you. Instead of eating all the wrong kinds of food, you eat the right kinds of food.

What you want to do is wake up those taste buds that were dulled (or murdered!) by all the salts and sweets that make up the junk food we eat. When you change the kind of foods you eat and begin to enjoy them, you'll find that your taste in food changes.

Instead of gulping your food, you can savor it. Instead of drowning it in sauces, creams, and dressings, you can enjoy each individual flavor. People with a healthy attitude toward food and who follow a healthy diet actually enjoy eating much more than people who swallow their food without tasting it.

This book doesn't contain menus or give specific information on calorie counting because there are many good books already on the market that provide such basic nutritional information. I urge you to buy a book that teaches about healthy foods.

Good nutrition and good health naturally go hand in hand. You can't have one without the other. Besides, life is not nearly as rewarding and full if you do not have good health. Do yourself a big favor, and eat healthy.

When you eat well-balanced, nutritious meals, you gain so much (not weight!). First, good eating naturally promotes a healthy weight. You aren't filling your body with empty calories that it can't use and only stores as fat. With the proper balance of foods, your body can process those calories and burn them efficiently. You'll also find yourself with more energy. With less weight to slow you down, you'll be able to move more freely and easily. You'll probably find that you can accomplish much more each day.

Good eating means you can sleep better. Your body heals more quickly from those minor cuts and bruises. You're better able to defend yourself against viruses and infections. People with poor eating habits battle not only with weight, but also chronic colds, coughs, and infections. By eating healthy you set yourself free from poor health.

Eating wisely and maintaining a healthy weight also helps you avoid more serious diseases such as diabetes, high blood pressure, and certain cancers. You give your heart and lungs a break, too. When you are overweight and not eating properly, every cell in your body is overtaxed. You become tired very easily.

Developing the right eating habits helps ensure that every cell and organ in your body can function at its best level. That means you can function at your best, too. That is what any diet should be about. Thin may be in, but there is much more to good health than just being thin. Whole people are healthy people with the confidence, strength, and energy to face any challenge of life and win!

Chapter 6

Here's Looking at You

Human improvement is from within outward.

—James Anthony Froude

Striving for good health is one of the greatest gifts we can give ourselves. It is difficult to achieve what we want in life if we let our health suffer needlessly. We never lose when we put some thought and effort into being healthy.

But if we are honest, we have to say that we don't always try to lose weight because of health. Often the desire to lose weight deals more with our looks than with our health. We want to look better because it is one way we can feel better about ourselves.

There is nothing wrong with wanting to look our best. In fact, that is something we all should strive for. Too often, among some Christians in the Church, the desire to be attractive has been viewed as vain or prideful and considered a sin. But I believe that God loves beauty and doesn't have a problem with us wanting to look as good as we can.

It is possible to put too much emphasis on physical beauty, however. If too much time, effort, energy, money, and thought are wrapped up in our looks, then we may find ourselves out of balance. That is where the danger of eating disorders such as anorexia sometimes develops. It can be dangerous to be obsessed with our looks.

We said in the previous chapter that the physical part of us must be balanced with all the other parts of us. The same is true with our looks as well as our health. Beauty is more than a flawless complexion, the perfect weight, the perfect height, or well-developed muscles. Beauty is something that arises from within us.

You have probably known someone who had a pretty face but an ugly personality. Your overall impression of that person was not favorable. Outer beauty cannot make up for a lack of beauty inside. That is why you must strive for wholeness in your life. Work on the inner qualities with as much diligence as you work on the outer qualities. Then you can be a truly attractive person.

True Beauty

There are probably as many explanations for what makes a person beautiful or attractive as there are people—and that's good. We are all unique and there is no reason we should be exactly like someone else. The old saying goes, "If you want to be an original, be yourself."

Just as deciding what weight is healthy for you is your choice, so is deciding what weight is the most attractive for you. If you don't agree with the idea that only skinny people are beautiful, then you may not be seeking to be a skinny person.

Image is not everything, though the media often implies that it is. Still, we all have to face the fact that we sometimes are judged by how we look. First impressions especially are often based upon one's physical appearance. That isn't necessarily right, but it does seem to be a fact of life.

This fact alone can put tremendous pressure on us to conform to the media's standard of beauty. I believe teens are particularly vulnerable to this kind of pressure, but we all must deal with it in some way or another. The question is, should the people who are trying to sell detergent, beer or cars have the final say about what is the right physical appearance for us? No! Yet, so often that is what we let happen.

Your goal is to look your best, not to look like the hottest fashion model, movie star, or rock musician. You are, or have the potential to be, just as attractive as anyone. How you look and how you feel about your looks is up to you. That means making decisions about what is right for you. Is it important to you to have a certain look? Is being beautiful an important goal for you? Only you can decide these things. Only you know how much emphasis you want to place on physical beauty.

Just remember, good looks are more than skin deep. Beauty is as much a part of your attitudes and actions as it is a part of your appearance. You can work to improve your looks—and we all should—but make them a part of the whole package. Look good, feel good, do good, be good. These things take effort on the inside as well as the outside.

If you like yourself, that attitude will be reflected in your looks. Self-confidence is a great beauty booster. Others are attracted to people who feel good about themselves. That's why it is so important to work on your thoughts at the same time you are working on your thighs. You will be beautiful when you think and act beautiful. The way you look tells the world how you feel about yourself.

Looking Good

Good looks are simply a combination of good health and good grooming. Anytime you work to improve your health, you automatically bring an improvement in your looks.

There are plenty of cosmetic companies that claim to sell beautiful, youthful looks from a bottle or a jar.

But all that any of them can offer is a copy of what nature itself provides through good health. Also, since so much of good health deals with good eating, you can, in fact, eat your way to better looks.

That's why striving to lose weight should always be done through an improvement in your eating habits. Crash diets seldom work because they are not based on healthy concepts. You might lose weight for a time, but if your health does not improve, chances are your looks won't improve either. You will end up dissatisfied with the results, and even may turn right around and gain back all the weight.

Consider some of the ways where improving your eating habits also improve your health and your looks.

1. Eating foods that are lower in calories means eating fruits, vegetables, and grains, all of which contain necessary vitamins and minerals. These are the basic ingredients that produce better health. Vitamins and minerals also promote clearer skin, shinier hair, and stronger teeth and nails, to name just a few of the benefits.

2. Eating foods that provide fiber also aids in the digestive process. Nutrients get into the bloodstream faster and toxins are flushed from the body more quickly. This keeps your skin glowing with a healthy look instead of becoming dull and yellowed.

3. Avoiding fats, cholesterol, and empty calories (such as those found in alcohol) makes less work for your body. You aren't wasting your body's time trying to process calories it can't use. Your blood will flow more freely, your liver functions more efficiently, and the pounds stay off. All of these things will produce a visible outward effect of health and beauty.

4. Drinking plenty of water is one of the simplest and most effective health and beauty aids. We are, of course, talking about purified or mineral water, not tap water. According to Rae Tyson in *USA Today* (9/27/93), a recent report by the Natural Resources Defense Council shows that 120 million people across America may be "needlessly exposed to unhealthy drinking water." In an analysis of EPA records, the Natural Resources Defense Council found that in 1991-92, 43 percent of all water supplies violated federal health standards. It seems that public drinking water can no longer be trusted.

You should try to get eight glasses of water (good water) a day. Water is the perfect diet drink—it has no calories! It also helps cut down your appetite. Water even helps burn stored fat, which produces energy.

Water is a vital lubricant for every cell in your body. It allows your joints and eyes to move more freely, and that helps combat arthritis. It increases the fluids in your blood and makes it flow faster. Best of all, water helps you look younger because it is a natural moisturizer and has a hydrating effect that gives your skin a smoother, softer texture.

Good looks are an inside job just like good attitudes or good actions. What you put into your body decides how your body looks and functions.

However, good looks are an outside job as well. Nothing will take the place of being healthy, but there are other ways you can enhance your looks. Good grooming is one way. No one will know you are healthy, strong, and beautiful if you sabotage your looks with sloppy, careless grooming.

Beauty and fitness are enhanced by the way you dress, the way you walk, and the way you present yourself. One of the added benefits of losing weight is a much wider range of choice in clothing. I've heard many people express the pleasure they felt in being able to wear attractive, well-fitting clothes after they lost weight. You look better when your clothes fit nicely.

Health and hygiene go hand in hand. Take the time necessary to keeping your body, your hair, and your clothes clean and looking their best. Think of good grooming as the attractive packaging of a great product—you!

Choices and Changes

Someone has said, "Choice, not chance, determines destiny." You don't have much control over the physical features you were born with, but that needn't stop you from making the best of them. If you are not happy with your appearance at age 20, you can blame nature. But if you aren't happy with your appearance at age 40, you have no one to blame but yourself.

Every human being comes in a unique, individual package. We are all just a bundle of possibilities. We must choose how we will think, feel, behave, and even look.

In the first chapter we talked about a woman named Marcie who grew up feeling badly about herself. She didn't think she was pretty and the extra weight she put on simply confirmed her thinking. Marcie finally had to face her thoughts and her weight and change both of them. She stopped slumping, stood up straight, changed her hairstyle, and took off 30 pounds. Now she feels good about herself and her looks. That gives her the confidence to face whatever situation life brings her way.

I don't know of anyone who doesn't go through times when they feel unattractive. When you reach that point, no matter what your age, you come to a place where you must make some choices. Will you use food as a comfort or as an excuse? Or will you control your thoughts, your emotions, and your eating habits?

Feeling attractive and being attractive are just two more choices we need to make for ourselves. How you look and how you feel about your looks can be determined by most of the things we have already discussed in this book. It's a mental and emotional matter as much as a physical matter. But let's look now at some of the choices we make that deal with the physical aspect of good looks.

Life Style

You may not think your life style has much to do with your physical appearance, but it plays a very vital role. How you choose to spend your time, money, and energy has a telling effect upon your body. If you are mistreating your body with an unhealthy life style, don't expect it to repay you by looking great.

The way we live determines how well we live and how long we live. If you're seeking a long, happy, healthy life, choose a wise life style. Don't expend your time, money, and energy on things that are frivolous, unimportant, or damaging to your health. Your body goes with you wherever you go for as long as you live. It would be smart to live in such a way that you and your body can be happy with each other for the rest of your life.

Work

A very important part of our life style is our work. We spend most of our adult life working at something. The choices you make in how and where you work also affect your body. The most important decision you make about taking a job might not be in terms of how much money you make, but how it affects your health.

There seems to be as many health hazards in today's business and industry as there were when the industrial revolution first began. These hazards are very different in our modern, high-tech era, but they still exist. You need to consider all these hazards when you make choices about your job.

Our work is also a main source of stress these days. A certain amount of stress can be good for us; it pushes us to perform our best. But too much stress can be another health hazard. Overeating is often related to the level of stress we endure. Stress can cause stomach and heart problems, and can contribute to those extra pounds, extra wrinkles, and extra gray hairs.

If you are experiencing such stress on your job that it affects your health, you need to make some choices, Look for the sources of the stress. Is the stress coming from pressures on the outside or are you putting pressure on yourself? Is there a way you can reduce it? Don't wait too long to do something about undue stress or your body might decide for you and break under the strain.

Recreation

Taking time out for play is one good way to relieve stress. I am a firm believer in the need for recreation—a time to get away from the everyday stresses and struggles and relax.

It doesn't have to be an expensive vacation to the Bahamas. It might be a simple backyard barbecue or a picnic in a park. Recreation is a way to restore our vitality and energy. When we've taken some time away from the job, we can usually go back to it with a renewed interest and zeal.

Taking the time to play gives your body a rejuvenating boost. Even a walk during your lunch break could make a vast difference in how well your day goes. Our bodies function best when we mix work with play. We feel and look better if we've taken the time to relax and enjoy life.

Rest

Closely tied with recreation is our need for rest. It wasn't an accident or afterthought that God designed the seven-day week to have in it one day for rest. He knew that we would need time off from work, time to catch up with sleep, and time to be quiet and reflective.

Different people need different amounts of sleep each day. Some can do quite well on only five or six hours; others need a full eight hours of sleep in order to function at their best. Decide how much you need and then set up your daily schedule to accommodate that need. Listen to what your body is telling you. If you always feel tired, you might not be getting enough sleep.

It may sound funny to call sleep your "beauty rest," but that's what it is in many ways. A good night's rest helps restore your body to its highest energy level. There's nothing attractive about dark circles under your eyes. Sleep helps you avoid such problems.

You also want to avoid eating a heavy meal late in the day because that can disrupt your sleep. Tossing and turning all night long isn't very restful. Don't carry your problems to bed either. Give them to God. He's going to be up all night anyway.

Exercise

The importance of exercise to health, fitness, and beauty cannot be overemphasized. We were created to be active, not to be couch potatoes. An exercise regimen of only two or three hours a week can make a vast difference in your life.

When Carl reached his fortieth birthday, he realized the pounds were creeping up on him. He wasn't interested in going on a strict diet, but he knew he needed to make some changes before the weight became a health problem. In analyzing his life style, he realized that he wasn't getting much exercise. So he set up an exercise program for himself that involved walking, swimming, and racquetball.

Within two weeks he noticed a difference in himself. By the time a month had passed, he had returned to his college weight and was feeling better than he had in years. To his surprise, he found that he was actually eating less. These many benefits came from only two hours of exercise per week.

Everyone knows exercise is good for them, but not everyone does something about it. Too often exercise seems like hard work. It's difficult to find the time; you have to buy special clothes or equipment; and it's just too hard to get started.

If you're one of those "I know I should, but I can't find the time" people, sit down and give exercise some thought. When you consider all the benefits that come from it, I think you'll find yourself more motivated to do it.

Start with something simple, like walking. Nearly everyone can walk. It doesn't take much time and it doesn't require special equipment; only a good pair of comfortable shoes. Even 30 minutes of walking per week can bring benefits. Once you begin, you'll find you enjoy it so much, it won't be hard to extend your exercise time.

Get involved with activities that you enjoy. If you've tried a certain form of exercise and didn't like it, then try something else. Don't give up. Even something like gardening can have exercise value.

Here are just a few of the exercises you could choose:

walking	tennis
jogging	racquetball
hiking	volleyball
biking	softball
rope jumping	basketball
swimming	aerobics

Consider exercise a reward that you give yourself. Learn to look forward to it. Enjoy the freedom, the movement, the strength, and the agility it brings. Then look in the mirror. You'll see a healthier, more attractive person looking back.

Exercise tones muscles, reduces flab, burns calories, cuts down on your appetite, reduces stress, increases circulation and lung capacity—the list can go on and on. After consulting your doctor about what's best for you, why not start an exercise program this week?

Habits

When the phone rang, George found himself reaching in two directions. One was to pick up the phone, the other was to grab a handful of jelly beans from the jar sitting on his desk. He did it automatically, without thinking about it.

"Do you always do that?" his friend Larry asked when George had finished his phone conversation.

"Do what?" George asked.

"Grab a handful of jelly beans every time the phone rings."

George frowned. "I don't know," he said. "I guess so. It's just a habit I picked up. I used to light up a cigarette but since I've quit smoking, I have to do something else. So I eat jelly beans."

"That might explain it, then," Larry said.

"Explain what?" George asked again.

"Before the phone rang, you were saying you'd put on a few pounds and you didn't know where they came from. I guess it's all those jelly beans."

George stared at the jar of brightly colored candy as if seeing it for the first time. Then he picked up the jar, crossed his office to the door, and stepped out to where his secretary sat. He placed the jelly beans on her desk.

"Here, Janet," he said. "Have some jelly beans."

Habits, as George discovered, can creep up on you without your realization. We might be surprised at what secret culprits are causing problems for our weight, our health, our looks.

Habits such as smoking are obvious problems. Everyone who smokes knows—even if they are unwilling to admit it—that the habit is bad for them. But giving it up is not easy. If you struggle with the habit—or addiction—of tobacco use, get some help in getting rid of it. You'll reap a multitude of benefits from such a victory.

The problems that smoking causes our health are well documented. However, most of us don't think much about the problems smoking can cause our looks. Cigarettes stain our hands, the ashes burn holes in our clothing, and the smoke increases wrinkling and irritation to our skin and eyes. In these days, smoking can be a big "turn off" to other people.

Some people say they don't want to quit smoking because they fear they will gain weight, and isn't that a health hazard too? Yet doctors say that someone who gives up smoking could gain as much as 30 pounds and still be healthier than if he continued smoking. Doctors further contend that the average person who gives up smoking gains no more than five to ten pounds, which is what most of us gain over the holidays. Even with some weight gain, a person will be healthier without tobacco.

Bad eating habits probably contribute to weight problems more than we realize. How easy it is to reach for food while we are watching television, reading a book, or talking on the phone. Most people snack not because they are hungry, but because it is a habit. When we break these habits, we take back the control over our weight and gain instead the benefits of being healthier and more attractive.

Check out your habits. Do you bite your nails? They won't be very attractive if you keep them bitten to the quick. Must you have a bedtime snack each night? How many unburned calories does that add to your weight? Do you drive everywhere you go when you could just as easily walk to some places? Save your car's energy and burn some of your own, and you'll be better off in several ways.

How easily our habits become necessities to us. That's why they seem so hard to break at times. But with a conscious effort, we can break any habit. Replace the bad habits with good ones.

Desires

What are your desires in life? Sometimes the things we want are not what is best for us. Sometimes they are things we cannot achieve. It's wonderful to have goals and aspirations—everyone should—but they must be attainable. If they aren't, you need to examine them honestly and then make any needed changes.

It would be a good thing for all of us to now and then re-check our lives and look for things that got out of balance or need to be changed. What desires must we lose because they are unhealthy, unproductive, or unrealistic? After we have decided what must be changed, then we must cultivate new desires of what to eat, what to think, and what to do.

Create the desires that are best for you. Desire health, strength, freedom, and control over your life. These are the things you can attain. Seek new desires and new habits in your eating, in your grooming, and in your thinking and attitudes. That is the way to win. That is the way to become the very best person you can be.

Social

Chapter 7

Avoiding the Social Traps

No man in the world has more courage than the man who can stop after eating one peanut.

—Channing Pollock

When was the last time you went to a social gathering where food was not served? If you're like me, it's hard to remember such an occasion. Food is almost always a part of social events. We get together, we talk and we laugh, we have a good time, and we eat!

In fact, food is so much a part of our social consciousness that the most important list a hostess makes is not the guest list, it's the grocery list. We often judge the success or failure of an event by its food.

When you're on a diet and trying to control what you eat, it can seem as though the entire world is geared toward food. Everywhere you turn, it's there to tempt you. It flickers across the television screen and stares up at you from magazine ads. It beckons from billboards and invites from store displays. You just can't get away from food.

But if you want to successfully control your weight and the importance of food in your life, you must deal with the social aspects of food and dieting. It doesn't have to overwhelm you. With the right plan, you can avoid the social traps that stand between you and the slimmer, healthier, more attractive you that you want to become.

In Temptation's Way

Since fast food and restaurants are a major industry in America, it's not surprising that we must face advertising of food everywhere. The result of so much emphasis on food is its apparent domination in our culture. Here in America, we have borrowed the recipes of the world. We can find just about any kind of food there is within easy reach.

When the whole country is having a love affair with food, is it any wonder that the majority of its people, at one time or another, struggle with a weight problem? Eating has become so convenient, easy, and inviting that it is difficult to resist such temptation.

You're sitting in front of the television munching on unbuttered popcorn—or your favorite, celery sticks—and an advertisement for pizza, fried chicken, or ice cream comes on. Suddenly you feel deprived and unloved. What's the point of being good? Why can't you eat that and still be thin, healthy, and happy? Self-pity is never far behind such thoughts and then, if you are not careful, self-indulgence follows.

You've finished lunch at a nice restaurant and you're feeling good about yourself because you chose your meal wisely. But then the dessert cart arrives. Everyone else at the table is making a selection and they urge you to do the same. If you take a slice of cheesecake, you'll feel guilty, but if you don't, you'll feel left out. Neither seems to be a choice you want to make.

You're going through the buffet at the office Christmas party. You've chosen a diet soda and have filled your plate with plenty of vegetables and some shrimp. But then you come to the cheese ball, and oh, goodness, someone brought a pecan pie. It is the holidays, you rationalize. They come only once a year. It won't hurt, just this once.

Don't think you are weak or a failure if you are vulnerable to the constant presence and availability of food in our society today. We've probably all found ourselves buying something to eat that we never intended to, simply because it was presented in an irresistible way.

If we indulged only once in a while, there might not be any harm in it. The idea behind establishing a healthy diet makes allowances for those occasional indulgences. The trouble is, "just this once" can easily become a regular habit and then we find that we have lost the battle.

Fighting With Temptation

Dieting would be so much simpler if all that food would just go away. But since that isn't likely, we must learn to deal with the temptation.

In the Bible, the apostle Paul had some advice for dealing with temptation. He said, "Flee!" (1 Tim. 6:11) It may seem cowardly to run away from tempting situations, but it is actually wise. You don't have to literally get up and run when the dessert cart comes by, but you can learn to avoid the places and situations that cause problems for you. As you grow stronger in your self-control, you can then face these situations and conquer them.

If a particular restaurant offers an entree that is your favorite, but not the wisest menu choice, you may want to stay away from that restaurant for a while. If those commercials on television make you feel deprived, change the channel! Walk away from the buffet table when you've filled your plate with all the foods that are good for you. Don't stand by the food all evening! Circulate and keep out of its reach as much as possible. Feast on good company and good conversation instead.

If the images of food in advertisements leave you feeling weak and vulnerable, try replacing them with good images. Cut out attractive, appetizing photographs of the foods that are good for you. That way you will be creating the desire for the right foods within you. When hunger strikes, you'll be hungry for foods that are healthy and beneficial.

As we said in Chapter 5, don't stock your kitchen with temptation. Buy the kinds of food that you can eat and leave the rest on the grocery shelves. The best way to resist temptation is to avoid it as much as possible.

Cultural Realities

People around the country and around the world pursue many different life styles. We are surrounded by certain traditions, certain ways of thinking, and certain ways of doing things. It is true for food as well as for other aspects of life.

Different areas of the country are known for their foods: Boston baked beans, Chicago deep-dish pizza,

Maine lobster, Southern fried chicken, Texas barbecue. You probably grew up enjoying traditional recipes or regional specialities, and these are a part of your life. They have a meaning and value far beyond their nutrition or calorie content.

As an evangelist, I travel throughout the United States and Europe. I've found that my hosts often are anxious to share with me some special food from their part of the world. Food is very much a part of the cultural landscape of a particular region.

America is known for its fast food. In Britain, I found that meat and potatoes were a staple at every meal. It was meat and potatoes or potatoes and meat. They couldn't imagine a meal without those two necessities. In Europe, bread and beer were prevalent at most meals. I noticed also that Europeans have a problem with weight just as Americans do.

Everywhere I go, I find people are always urging me to eat. "Try some of this. How about some of that?" Since I try to be careful about what I eat, I've learned to say no as tactfully, but as firmly, as possible. Some people can be quite insistent or easily hurt if you're not interested in eating their food.

You may encounter this problem also as you work on changing your eating habits. When certain foods are a part of our cultural identity, it can be difficult to give up those foods or eat less of them. When they are served as a form of hospitality, it may be even more difficult to refuse them.

Probably the one time—besides the holidays—when your diet is hardest to maintain is your vacation. When you are visiting new places, it's only natural to want to taste the local cuisine. And you should at least sample some of the foods that are available in the places you travel. Learning about other cultures involves learning about their food. But let moderation be the key when you are sampling new foods.

If you can't refuse what is being offered, yet it doesn't fit well into your healthier diet, try limiting the amount you eat. As you travel, identify the foods in the area that are healthy and low in calories, and make those the foods you sample most.

Staying at home presents challenges as well in eating foods that have cultural significance. Almost every family has traditional foods that are a part of its heritage. For some reason, the most healthy and nutritious foods aren't always the ones that become traditions.

For those traditional dishes that have been handed down through the generations, you might try modifying the recipes. Substitute healthier ingredients for those that are high in fat and cholesterol. You might come up with something just as delicious and far more nutritious than what you've been eating. You may even start a tradition of your own.

Social Scene

At the beginning of the chapter we noted that nearly all social events include food. If you go to a ball game, there are peanuts, hot dogs, beer, pretzels, and dozens of other foods. At the movie theater, you can munch on candy, popcorn, and other sticky items. Parties always include food, and plenty of it. Banquets and board meetings, even budget planning sessions, offer us something to eat.

The banquet circuit has been the downfall for many a professional athlete. After they retire from sports, they often go on the speaking circuit. Almost always they speak at a banquet. The weight goes on fast because they are no longer as active, but continue eating as if they were. Look at all those coaches, managers, and sports announcers who advertise for diet drinks. Most of them are retired athletes who forgot to stop eating as if they were still out on the playing field.

Putting on weight became a hazard of their new careers. Putting on weight may seem like a hazard on your job as well. If your work entails many social gatherings or meetings, chances are you are eating as you work.

In such situations, there can be a tremendous amount of pressure placed upon you to eat. The pressure may be subtle. It might only be from a hostess wanting to be sure you are enjoying yourself. Nevertheless, that kind of pressure is real.

Shirley had a job in public relations that required her attendance at a number of social events. She was invited to a dinner attended by many big movie stars, politicians, and sports figures. Her husband was supposed to go with her, but just before they were to leave the house, they had a serious argument and he refused to go.

Shirley went on to the party because her job required it, but she was miserable the whole time. She parked herself in front of the buffet table and nibbled all evening. She met some interesting people and made some important contacts, but she also gained a few unnecessary pounds.

This can be the problem that many of us face. Emotional strains are compounded by the fact that we are social creatures who must go out and face the world—and food—even while we are dealing with things difficult for us. Those moments when we are particularly vulnerable to the temptation of food somehow seem to come just when we must attend some social function where food is served.

That is why it is so important to understand our emotions and the role they play in our eating. We can't ask the world to stop pushing food at us while we have a pity party or deal with something more serious. The temptation will always be there. We must learn how to overcome it.

First you need to recognize how much of your eating is a part of your social life. Do you go out to lunch each day with a group from the office? Perhaps you are eating a noon meal whether or not you are hungry simply because you want the company of your fellow workers. I'm not saying there is something wrong with eating lunch with friends; just be aware of this eating habit.

If you're not hungry, don't be afraid to say no. Most people will understand that. If you feel comfortable with telling your friends that you are trying to lose weight, go ahead and say it. You might be surprised at how supportive they will be. You'll probably learn that many of your friends are trying to lose weight, too. You can help each other.

Be conscious of what you order in a restaurant on these luncheon outings. If everyone else is having the same thing, but you feel it would not be a healthy choice for you, then stand your ground and order what you think is best. Don't go along with the crowd.

One easy way to cut calories at restaurant meals is to drink water instead of a soft drink. Ask for bottled water if its available and you prefer its taste, or ask for a lemon wedge to give regular water a better flavor. Also, many menus these days offer light items. One of those might be a good choice for you.

Or choose a salad, fresh fruits, or vegetable dishes—all can be wise, healthy choices as long as you stay away from heavy dressings, sauces, or creams.

Don't eat because someone else wants you to eat. Well-meaning friends may urge you to try something new, to take a second helping, or to have some dessert. It's okay to say no. You can be polite, but firm, and usually they will get the message.

Another hazard to diets that many Christians face is the after-church fellowship. It's quite a common practice for a group of friends to go out to eat after a service. This is especially dangerous if you're having a special week of services! You can put on ten pounds by the time the meetings are through.

I sometimes think it is all the "fellowshipping" we do that results in so many "wide-body" ministers, for in Christian circles, fellowshipping usually means food! If a minister is expected to participate in the fellowship, he faces the difficult task of being diplomatic about refusing some of Sister Higgenbothom's peach pie.

I'm not in any way suggesting that we should do away with the fellowship. I'm not even suggesting we do away with the food of the fellowship. But the food should be balanced with other things. Laughter, love, caring, sharing, and growing (not physically!) should be the most important parts of the time we spend with our brothers and sisters.

Be aware of your eating at these times of fellowship. It's easy to get caught up in the good time you are having and not notice how much food you are eating. The same rules for eating with the office lunch crowd apply here. Don't let a social setting be an excuse not to eat sensibly.

Overcoming the Pressures

It can be difficult to follow a healthy diet when everyone else is eating anything and everything they want. Sometimes diets are easier to follow when we are eating alone. There's less temptation and we feel more in control. Probably more diets are destroyed at social gatherings than in any other way.

When we think of peer pressure, we usually think of teenagers trying to cope with high school and college. But people in the work force know there is still pressure to follow the crowd even after the teen years. It can be much more subtle, but it is still real.

That is why you must be strong in yourself. Many forces outside you would undermine your resolve if you let them. But when you know within yourself what you want to be and what goals you are striving for, then you can overcome the temptations of the social scene. The battle may not be any easier, but the victory is more sure.

Just remember to:

1. Think healthy, positive thoughts.
2. Eat the right words and images.
3. Learn to love and accept yourself.
4. Practice healthy choices, positive attitudes, and proper control.
5. Set realistic goals with realistic deadlines and keep them in front of you.
6. Look out for yourself by planning ahead and staying away from temptation.

A boxer must weigh no more than the maximum amount of pounds allowed in order to stay in his weight class. He must take care of his body despite the publicity functions where food is served. He must be disciplined to keep his goal always before him. If he isn't disciplined, not only will he be overweight, but he'll also lose his next fight before he steps into the ring.

Think of yourself as a successful, healthy, happy individual in training for a big fight. The fight is for life itself, and you'll win if you have the discipline and strength to resist the temptation and pressures the social world holds.

Over the River and Through the Woods

If you are like most people, you heard a lot about starving children in India or Africa during mealtimes when you were a child. Parents used the "starving children in another part of the world" as a strong incentive to get you to clean your plate. If that didn't work, there was always the threat of "no dessert until you eat your vegetables."

Many adults today still feel guilty if they don't clean their plate at mealtimes. That is especially true if they are visiting their mothers.

We've already stated that you can't let the lessons of childhood rule you as an adult. You know very well that whether or not you eat won't help or hurt the starving children in India. It will harm you if you overeat all the time. But the "starving children guilt syndrome" still works in the mind of many people to eat, eat, eat.

The problem of eating to please our mothers is compounded by the fact that we often eat at Mom's during the holidays—a time when we are all prone to indulging ourselves just a bit. Thanksgiving and Christmas become a double hazard for those trying to be careful about what they eat and to maintain a healthy weight.

You go to your grandmother's or your mother's house to visit them and what do you hear? "Aren't you hungry? You hardly touched your plate. Don't you want a second helping? How about a little more apple pie." Mothers never stop being mothers even when their children have gray hair and grandchildren of their own. They are concerned about the well-being of their kids and they want to make sure they are eating enough.

Most of us are in little danger of not eating enough, but it's hard to convince some mothers of that. When I visited my mother during Hanukkah, all I heard was eat, eat, eat.

"What's the matter," she said. "Don't you eat three meals a day?"

"No, I don't eat three meals a day."

"Why don't you eat three meals a day?"

"Because I don't have to eat three meals a day."

I don't think she understood. Most people have it in their minds that everyone is supposed to eat three meals a day with a snack or two besides. That is in their minds, though; it's not in mine. Because it is not in my mind, I don't feel the need to eat a set amount of meals each day. You don't have to either.

But many people are afraid to say no—especially to a mother, grandmother, aunt, or some other relative. It can sometimes seem easier to keep the holidays peaceful and eat what is offered you.

The best way I know to deal with a relative who is pushing food at you is to be polite, honest, and firm. Usually, if you tell your family that you are limiting the amount of food you eat for the sake of your health, they will understand and be supportive. Mothers are always concerned about their children's health. Just be sure that your mother understands you are not implying that her cooking is bad for your health. You are limiting all foods—not just hers.

Holidays are supposed to be a wonderful time spent with family and friends. If your time with family is tense, upsetting, and frustrating, you may want to consider limiting the time you spend with them as well as limiting the amount of food you eat. If emotions are troubled by a visit back home, you are likely to eat even more than you intended. Be wise and careful about your holiday visits and everyone will have a healthier, happier time.

We all want to please the people we love. But sometimes we must say no to them and that can be difficult. I believe the people who truly love us will understand when we try to bring improvement to our lives. They want what is best for us. So we must have the strength and freedom to say, "No, thank you. I've had enough to eat for now."

Getting Along

Sometimes it may seem that we are walking a tightrope between pleasing others and pleasing ourselves. Someone else's ideas and our ideas about what is best for us might not always be the same. Then what do we do?

You will never be able to please everyone. Trying to do just that is what got many people into trouble, not just with their weight, but also in other areas. What usually happens is you end up pleasing no one, not even yourself.

If you put on 10 or 20 pounds because you can't say no to well-meaning friends, family, and hosts, they won't have to live with that. You will. Sooner or later you may come to regret and resent it. The anger that results probably won't help your efforts to slim down and could even cause problems for your relationships. It's better—though often harder—to do what you know is best for yourself, even if it means not conforming with the people around you.

Remember, you are the one who has to live with yourself. You have to walk around inside your body all the time. You have to look at yourself in the mirror. If you're not able to please everyone else, at least work at pleasing yourself. Make decisions that are right for you and that will help you reach the place you want to be.

They say that misery loves company, but it's also true that people who aren't miserable don't want to be around those who are. Thus, another reason to work at maintaining a weight you can feel good about is to keep you—and everyone around you—from being miserable. Losing weight should primarily be something you do for yourself, for health, or for other reasons. However, it doesn't hurt your relationships if you are a healthier, happier person. Neither does it hurt your social life. When you've become the person you want to be, you'll be someone whom others want to be around.

Chapter 8

Priority One

A man's interest in the word is only an overflow from his interest in himself.

—George Bernard Shaw

We all face pressures in social settings. The only way to deal with that pressure is to have already established our priorities in our own minds. As we have said, we'll never be able to please everyone. We probably won't even please ourselves all the time. But we can know what we want from life and we can work toward that goal regardless of what the world says or does.

We must know what our own convictions are. We've all heard the expression, "You have to stand for something or you will fall for anything." Society today has plenty of things that can trip us up. It's important for us to know where we are going and how we intend to get there so we won't stumble over the obstacles placed in our way.

The thoughts you think, the emotions you feel, and the actions you take will either give you victory or bring defeat. It's a matter of each individual "eating" the right words and finding the power behind those words. This is the key to victoriously facing all that life brings your way—even in dieting. You must have the power behind the words to stand up for your convictions. "I will not overeat. I will not gain unwanted weight. I will not compromise what I know is right for me."

Without that power you will give in to temptation. "Everyone else is eating, so I'll eat, too." Without convictions you are willing to stand for, the people and situations in your life that could be your greatest assets become your biggest downfall.

Finding a Fit

You need to take care of yourself. Now, I'm not advocating a "look out for number one" attitude. I think the greatest kind of life you can live is one like Jesus lived—one of helping others and giving of yourself. But if you're not healthy and whole, you won't be able to live that kind of life. That's why it is important for you to know what you want to be and then to work toward those goals. You need to take care of you. Only then will you truly be able to take care of someone else.

Sometimes following your convictions can make you feel like a salmon swimming upstream. It seems like a fight just to hold on to what you believe. The world always tries to squeeze you into its mold. But the Bible tells us not to be conformed to the world, but to be transformed by the renewing of our minds (Rom. 12:2). Make up your mind and then keep thinking the strong, positive thoughts that help you stay true to your beliefs.

Sure, it's hard to make the swim upstream alone. We are social creatures and need the companionship of other people. Therefore, it is important to make wise choices about fitting in with other people. We want to choose the right companions.

Proverbs 13:20 says, "He that walketh with wise men shall be wise: but a companion of fools shall be destroyed." In some way or another, you become like the people who are a part of your life. They influence you and you influence them. The more time you spend with certain people, the more likely you are to follow them in the choices and actions they make.

If you've chosen wisely, their influence will be good. Your friends should help you to be your best. "Iron sharpeneth iron;" the Bible says, "so a man sharpeneth the countenance of his friend" (Prov. 27:17). Two strong, healthy people can combine in friendship and love to bring out the best in each other. When you find a relationship like that, it is very special and should be highly valued.

Not all the people you live with, work with, and know will bring out your best, however. Any friend who says to you, "Let's get high; let's get drunk; or let's pig out," is a dubious friend. Such friends will lead you in a direction that will neither benefit you nor bring about the desired result of being healthy and whole.

That is why Proverbs also advises, "Be not among winebibbers; among riotous eaters of flesh: for the drunkard and the glutton shall come to poverty: and drowsiness shall clothe a man with rags" (Prov. 23:20-21). Trying to fit in with the "party crowd" can have consequences that undermine your efforts to be a successful, healthy individual.

I'm not saying we can't get together with friends and have a good time. Friendship should be fun as well as serious. But we must know what kind of fit we are looking for when it comes to friendship. The crowd we choose to fit in with may determine how well everything else fits in our lives. If we fit in with the wrong people, we may not be able to fit into our clothes!

Complainer or Champion?

Judy had moved to a new city and was trying to start her life over after a divorce. She knew very few people in her new location and felt lonely and scared. When a fellow worker invited her to a party, she thought it would be a good way to make friends.

She met several friendly people and soon was receiving more invitations to social events. She had been accepted into the group and at first it felt good to her. But she slowly began to realize that "the gang," as they called themselves, were monopolizing all her time. They also expected her to go along with everything they did.

Judy didn't feel comfortable with some of the choices "the gang" made, but she was afraid to speak up for herself. She was afraid that if she refused to do something with them, they would stop inviting her and reject her.

Rejection was something Judy feared and the pressure she felt from this social situation became her excuse to eat. Instead of feeling better about herself, though, she just felt worse and worse.

Then a neighbor invited her to a church service. Judy had always attended church back in her hometown, but she had stopped when she moved. That church service made her face what she had been doing to herself. She realized that she had made some wrong choices. Judy knew she had to get hold of herself and stand on her convictions.

As Judy expected, "the gang" lost interest in her because she no longer went along with every decision they made. But by that time Judy was making new friends at church. She felt better about herself, she was more in control of her emotions and her actions, and without even consciously dieting, she came back to a healthy weight.

What's more, Judy found she wasn't complaining all the time anymore. Her old friends had found it fashionable to criticize and complain about everything. In general, though they laughed a lot, "the gang" had been a very negative group. Judy had been influenced by that negative attitude and only as she pulled away from their influence did she see how destructive her friendship with them had been.

We might be accepted by the party crowd, but if that acceptance brings negative feelings and actions instead of positive ones, we're not doing ourselves any favors. Nothing can make us feel guilty any faster than the realization that we have betrayed our own inner convictions.

You must live with you. If a relationship is tearing you up inside, something has to change. You don't have to abandon your friends, but you must decide at some time that you will no longer compromise what you believe to be right for you. That decision can result in some "friends" abandoning you. I wish that weren't true, but it does happen. Rejection always hurts, but in the long run, you will be much better off.

Why be friends with someone or why hang around with a group that only makes you feel badly about yourself? You will end up being a complainer instead of a champion.

Sometimes it is as important to know where you don't fit in as it is to know where you do fit in. The wrong crowd can be so hurtful. There is no reason why you should belong to the most "in" group of people. Find a place where you can be comfortable, where you can be your best. Don't compromise on this; it's too important.

How much do you love yourself? How much do you want to take care of yourself? Do you want to be one of those complainers? Or do you want to be one of the champions—those who have the determination to stand for themselves and be their best?

Right and Wrong Desires

I don't think most of us realize what a vital role the people in our lives play in determining our desires. You may be reading this book right now because someone dropped the hint that you need to lose a little weight. Even subtle hints from people we care about can have a big impact on how we think and behave.

If this were an ideal world, then our friends and family would influence us to do only good things and to have only the right desires. But this is an imperfect world and sometimes the people who inhabit it don't have our best interests at heart. They can lead us to the wrong desires, and that can lead to destructive decisions.

Before I became a Christian, I used to take drugs—all kinds of drugs. My friends did drugs, too. But I grew very dissatisfied with that kind of life and began looking for something else. I began to search for God. The hungrier I became for spiritual things, the less I desired drugs. When I made Jesus my friend, He healed me of all the effects of drugs and I've never had a desire for them since.

It took me more than a year to find my way out of drugs and into a new life in Christ. Maybe if I had known someone who could help me in my search, I would have progressed much faster. But I had to make the journey alone. It was an uphill fight that I'm sure would have been simpler and easier if I had just had a friend to help me.

Today if someone were to offer me drugs, my answer would be a quick no. I've long since left behind all the friends I got high with, and now I "get high" on spiritual things with a new set of friends. My desires have completely changed.

If you've come to recognize that you have some desires that are unhealthy for you, now is the time to make a change. You can lose those wrong desires.

What are wrong desires? The Bible is the best place to start looking for answers to that question. So I won't give you a long list; I'll just say that a wrong desire is anything that would hurt you or someone else. If your desire for certain foods causes weight and health problems, then for you that is a wrong desire. It might not be wrong for someone else because it doesn't cause them the problems that it causes you. But for you, it just isn't healthy, wise, or right.

Are your friends encouraging the right desires in you, or the wrong ones? What is your reaction when someone says, "Let's get high; let's get drunk; or let's pig out"? Can you say no to people important to you because you know what they are asking is wrong? You'll have to find the strength to do that if you hope to be the best person you can be.

Life is just a series of choices. Some are big choices, some are little choices, but they all make a difference in our lives. Sometimes the choices that seem so small and insignificant later prove to be very important ones. Therefore we can't get lazy, take things for granted, or let down our guard. What we decide today will make a difference tomorrow.

You can change your desires. Sometimes it may seem impossible, but you can. The best way to lose a wrong desire is to replace it with a good one. If you crave too much of the wrong kinds of food, cultivate an appetite for healthier foods. It's just a matter of revamping your mind: thinking differently, acting differently, reacting differently.

When you are in control of the choices you make—instead of just going along with others—then you feel better about yourself. You feel more confident and you can make the changes you want. Confidence in one area can also help in every other area of your life. So know when to say when. Know when to say no.

Keeping Up With the Joneses

Sometimes our desires are driven by a sense of competition or a need to feel that we measure up to others. If you've ever found yourself buying something or trying something just to keep up with a friend, fellow worker, or neighbor, then you know about this kind of desire.

Probably half the diets begun in this world are started because we can't let someone else look better in a swimsuit than we do. Competition can be healthy and fun, but like everything else in life, it must be balanced with common sense and reality. Keeping up with the Joneses is a stupid reason to kill ourselves with overwork or an unhealthy diet.

Kathleen was always on a diet, although she didn't need to be. She was not overweight; she was just insecure about her looks. She was always looking enviously at other women and feeling that she didn't measure up. When she would see someone she thought was beautiful and successful, she would dive into another diet, hoping that it would magically make her beautiful and successful. All it ever did was make her miserable.

Kathleen is still dieting today, even though people are always saying to her, "You don't need to diet. You look great the way you are." She doesn't believe them. She thinks they are just being nice. So every time she flips through a magazine, she believes that she isn't as attractive as she should be. Kathleen has let envy and jealousy steal her enjoyment of life. She needs to learn to like herself and value the special person that she is.

Are you jealous of those skinny people in the magazine ads? Do you feel that life has been unfair to you because you have not been blessed with the perfect body, the perfect house, car, job, and spouse—even the perfect life? Is that your motivation for starving yourself, working two jobs, or spending more money than you make?

Jealousy of others steals your happiness and creates bitterness, anger, and suspicion. It's a waste of your emotional energy. Spend your emotions on feeling good about what you do have and what you already are. Of course you can work toward more and better things in your life. It's good to have goals. But don't let jealousy drive your desires and determine the actions you take.

If you look around, you will always find someone who is more fortunate than you. But keep looking. There are others who are less fortunate than you. Is being as thin, as rich, or as fashionable as someone else really that important? Striving for what is healthy—even if it's different from "the Joneses"—is what counts.

Active and Involved

Some of the happiest and most satisfied people I know are my older friends and acquaintances who have gotten past all that "rat race" competition and learned to savor the truly important things of life. I guess wisdom does come with age because it seems that they have found the secret to a successful life.

I've never met an elderly person who was on a diet or who worried about buying the latest fad. Sure, older people have concerns. Life doesn't get easier as we get older, but we do seem to handle it better. Maybe we should pay more attention to our elders and see if we can learn some things from them that we can put to use while we are still young.

Once I was visiting with an elderly gentleman who is a greeter at Wal-Mart. He always has a friendly smile and is eager to help the customers who come into the store. I know his smile comes from more than just doing his job because no one can fake the cheerful attitude he always has.

I asked my friend why he hadn't retired by now. He said he liked to stay active and involved and didn't want to waste away at home doing nothing. Helping people gave him a good feeling and that contributed to his alertness and his excellent health. He had no plans to retire.

There is something revitalizing about getting out of the house and being actively involved in life. Too often people who do not feel good about how they look tend to stay at home and hide. That only contributes to their negative feelings. It keeps the focus of their attention upon themselves and then they blow their flaws out of proportion.

There is a negative cycle that develops when you refuse to go out into public because of your weight or some other problem. When you avoid people and situations that might make you uncomfortable, you only reinforce your fears and insecurities. That makes it more and more difficult to get out into the world. It creates even more insecurity and self-doubt. It's a no-win situation.

Believe it or not, getting out and being active will help your self-esteem. Sure, you may run into situations that are new and perhaps a bit awkward at first. No one is born with perfect social skills. They have to be developed. The way you develop them is through practice, trial-and-error, and try, try, try again.

Don't wait until you are a perfect weight to live a full, active life. Always try new things, meet new people, and experience new situations. Each time you make an effort to get to know someone, to help someone who is less fortunate than you, to reach out beyond your own world, you become a better, more confident, more vital person. These experiences can be so helpful in feeling good about yourself. That, in turn, helps with the nitty-gritty work of losing weight or changing yourself in some other way.

But what if a person tries something new and he falls flat on his face? Wouldn't the humiliation drive a person even further into a protective shell? That is certainly a real possibility. It's simply a matter of choice, however. You can be so embarrassed in a social situation that you vow never to leave the house again. Or you can laugh at your mistake and go on with your life.

We all make mistakes. We've all put our foot in our mouth by saying the wrong thing at the wrong time. I don't know of anyone who hasn't done that at one time or another. If you make a mistake, chances are you will simply make everyone else feel more comfortable with you because they make mistakes too. Don't retreat into a shell because you slipped and fell.

Do you know that there are people who use their weight as a kind of shell to hide behind? I've been told by a friend of mine that she has chosen to remain overweight because she believes it will keep the men away from her. "I'm happily married," she told me. "I don't want to be tempted by someone else."

I think there are other ways to avoid such temptation. But my friend's weight is her choice and if she feels okay about it and it isn't causing her any health problems, then I'm not going to criticize her. But what about you? Do you hide behind a few extra pounds? Is it a way to keep people at a distance? I don't mean any pun by that. I'm sincerely asking you to consider whether you might not be having trouble losing weight because you really don't want to. Perhaps you are using it as a defense mechanism or as a protection against being hurt.

If that is the case, then you need to recognize it. You need to decide if you want things to stay that way. If you want to change, you can. Losing weight might be a risk, but it might also be the key to unlocking your potential and letting you become your best.

To Dare and Endure

The battle to better ourselves can seem like a time not only to dare to try new things, but also to endure some of the discomfort that change inevitably brings. That's why dieting, or any new discipline, takes strength and even a certain amount of courage. Change can be frightening, and we need the inner determination to follow through on what we have set out to do.

I remember a time several years ago during a fast. My fast was of a spiritual nature, rather than trying to lose weight, but it took determination just the same. While I was fasting some friends took me to a restaurant at the Mauna Kea Beach Hotel in Hawaii where I was living at the time.

That hotel offered one of the best buffets in the world. Several European chefs were employed there, each creating his own specialty. The first thing I would usually do when I went there was hit the dessert counter. They have the best desserts I've ever tasted anywhere, offering 25 different pastries as well as many other mouth-watering choices. But on that particular day, I was fasting and I didn't intend to break my fast.

My friend said, "Aren't you going to eat?"

I told him, "No."

"It's on me," he insisted.

"You go ahead and eat," I said.

That took determination. I had made a decision and even though it was a tough one to keep at that moment, I made the choice to deny myself and keep my fast. You will face similar choices as well if you have decided to live a life style that is healthy and balanced.

When it comes to living a very disciplined life, I think of a man like Mahatma Gandhi of India. He lived a fasted life and he did so because he was determined to fast for India. His inner convictions drove him to do what he felt he had to do for his people. He made the tough choices for his life, and they changed an entire nation.

But I don't want to paint a grim picture of a disciplined life. Every hurdle that you make over some obstacle strengthens you for the next one. That way the obstacles and temptations become easier to manage as you become stronger and more disciplined. Eventually this healthy, whole way of living becomes a pleasure.

You gain strength as you daily apply the principles you've learned here. This may mean denying yourself some things that are neither healthy nor the right choice for you. Following your inner convictions may lead you against the tide of popular opinion, but you must listen to what they tell you.

Being your best isn't a matter of keeping up with someone else. It takes knowing who you are and who you want to be—on the inside as well as the outside. Knowing where you are now and where you want to go with your life is half the battle in getting there.

Someone has said, "Success is a journey, not a destination." That is true of the whole, disciplined, healthy life that you want to live. You never arrive there; you are always traveling. But the journey can be a good one if you enjoy the company not only of good friends and family, but also of yourself.

Spiritual

Chapter 9

Wisdom and Practicality

Great men are they who see that the spiritual is stronger than any material force.

—Ralph Waldo Emerson

The spiritual nature of mankind is hard to define and often misunderstood. Many people ignore the spiritual part of their lives and thus never truly live a whole life. Just because we cannot see our spirits does not mean that they do not exist or are unimportant. The spirit is, in fact, the most important part of us.

Our spirit beings are the part of us that remain long after the body is gone. Since we live in the spirit realm for eternity and in the bodily realm for only a few years here on earth, it is just common sense to devote some care and attention to our spirits. The spirit has as much to do with health and wholeness as any other part of our beings.

What Is Spirituality?

The spirit is our true self; we only inhabit the body. The Bible sometimes refers to the body as a tent, a temple, or even an earthenware jar that holds the spirit. The body is important, but not more important than the spirit. The spirit is the inner, eternal part of us. It is invisible, yet very powerful. So far in this book we have dealt with the mind, the heart, and the body. Now we need to consider how the spirit plays an important part in our lives and health.

Being spiritual is more than just being religious. Many people are religious without ever understanding their spirits. For them religion is a ritual or a set of moral beliefs. It may provide them with direction, purpose, and comfort in their lives, but it doesn't move beyond the realm of their bodies and minds to touch the inner person.

While I was ministering in Europe last year, I met a minister who weighed more than 300 pounds. His eating habits were very poor and he apparently would eat anything put in front of him, since I watched him devour pickles dipped in marmalade.

This man thought he was very spiritual and enjoyed telling other people how to solve their problems.

However, it is my opinion that a person can't be truly spiritual and weigh 300 pounds. That isn't a healthy or an attractive weight for anyone. If we are spiritual, we will have the victory over the desires, thoughts, and emotions that cause us to overeat. Then we can lose the weight and get our lives in better order.

This minister's attitude was, "No one can tell me anything. I'm spiritual." I said to him, "Oh, yeah? Go look in the mirror." He just looked at me instead. He didn't understand what I was telling him.

Spirituality is not some pie-in-the-sky state of mind either. It is not just the part of us that is reserved for Heaven and useless for here and now. True spirituality is wisdom and practicality for coping with the challenges of life that we experience every day.

Our spirits should not be fed only on Sundays and ignored or starved through the rest of the week. It is such an essential part of us that without its life and strength working inside, we will never be whole people. Something will always be missing from our lives.

Spiritual Hunger

We evangelists like to say that within every individual is a God-shaped vacuum that only God can fill. Nothing else will fit in the place meant for God. Yet many people spend their entire lives trying to find something else to fill the void within them.

However, nothing but God will satisfy a hunger for God. Believe me, I know, for I tried many different things myself: money, drugs, women, fast cars, jetsetting with the stars. Yet none of these things satisfied me down inside my spirit. Then I made a New Year's resolution to try to find God and after a long search through my Old Testament, I finally did.

God is a Spirit, and He made us spirit beings. The way we can know God is through the spirit. But until we come to a place where we begin a relationship with the Lord, our spirits are like seeds that haven't been planted yet. The spirit has life within it, but that life is dormant.

Evangelicals use the term "born again" to describe what happens when the seed of the spirit bursts forth into new life at the time we come to God. We get this term from something Jesus said to Nicodemus, a religious leader who had come to Him with questions about what He was teaching. "Except a man be born again," Jesus said, "he cannot see the kingdom of God" (Jn. 3:3).

Our first birth is physical. We come into the world as little babies, after we have grown from two tiny seeds united in our mothers' womb. We are born again when our spirits are birthed by the Holy

Spirit of God. Only when we have found this new life will our spiritual hunger be satisfied.

Many people do not understand their spiritual hunger. They know they are hungry and they are dissatisfied with life as it is, but they don't know how to meet that spiritual need. Often they eat food, thinking they are physically hungry. But physical food doesn't satisfy a spiritual hunger. The desire for God, like the desire for love, cannot be satisfied by eating food.

Most of us have a desire to be married. We spend considerable time and energy looking for that special someone whose heart will join with ours in love. Until that person is found, though, we always feel that something is missing from our lives. It's the same way with God. Until we find Him, there is a piece missing from our lives. We can't be whole without God.

Philip was a brilliant musician and composer with degrees from several major music schools. His compositions had won him awards and acclaim, but it wasn't enough to satisfy him. He was always looking for some new and more challenging accomplishment to bring the fulfillment he desired.

Philip was working on the score for a movie and it was one of the most challenging compositions he had ever attempted. But a part of the movie dealt with the spiritual awakening of one of the characters. Philip found it difficult to write a piece of music that would fit the mood and meaning of that particular scene. It bothered him that he couldn't write this piece. He'd never had a problem before.

The longer he worked on it, the more frustrated he became. Then suddenly he realized he couldn't write the music because he had never experienced a spiritual awakening. He'd never even thought much about the spiritual part of himself.

At first his spiritual search was out of curiosity and a need to finish the music he was writing. But as his search took him to the Bible, he found a hunger growing within him that he knew would never be satisfied until he had found a relationship with God. He finally came to the point where he was ready to pray one of those old-fashioned prayers of repentance that lead to salvation. Philip was born again.

Now the music flowed out of him. He finished the score in record time. The piece that had once been so difficult was the best he had ever written. It began softly, like the awakening of spring, and trumpeted to a finale of joy, power, and life.

No matter how much we like to eat, we cannot get the joy, power, and triumph of the spirit through physical food. If we try to satisfy a spiritual hunger with food—no matter how wholesome and nutritious—we will probably just end up overeating and still feel hungry and dissatisfied. We must learn how to feed the inner part of us as well.

Feeding the Spirit

Between the time of my bar mitzvah when I was 13 years old and the time I began my spiritual search about ten years later, I didn't have much interest in religion or God. I didn't have the hunger for spiritual things. My tastes ran toward much more carnal values.

But when I did become hungry to know God, my tastes changed. The life I had been living no longer satisfied me. I craved things of a much more lasting value and quality.

Even my physical tastes changed after I became a Christian. I never used to like salads. Now I eat them all the time. I don't crave junk anymore; I look forward to a light meal of lean meats and crisp vegetables. When God changes you, He changes all of you for the better.

Feeding the spirit requires spiritual food. You can feed your spirit much the same way you feed your mind: with positive words and images from the Word of God. Remember, Proverbs 4:20-22 says, "My son, attend to my words; incline thine ear unto my sayings. Let them not depart from thine eyes; keep them in the midst of thine heart. For they are life unto those that find them, and health to all their flesh."

The spirit, like the mind, the heart, and the body, can be strong or weak. It can be healthy or unhealthy.

It can grow, develop, and change, or it can stay the same. It can be vital and alive or it can wither and die. Your spirit will be as strong and as healthy as you determine to make it—and that will depend upon how well you feed it.

I believe we all need to have a greater craving for spiritual things. The Bible is the best-selling book in the world, but it is probably one of the least read. It won't do your spirit any good if it sits on the shelf gathering dust. Your body wouldn't be healthy if you bought plenty of food but never ate any of it. Your spirit is the same way.

"But I don't understand the Bible and I find it boring." People who say that probably never had their spirits brought to life. The Bible is a spiritual book. The mind only understands part of it. To read and feed from the Word of God, you must have an open, living spirit.

"Thy words were found, and I did eat them; and Thy word was unto me the joy and rejoicing of mine heart" (Jer. 15:16a). Food is often used in the Bible to symbolize the Word's truth and teaching that give life and strength to the spirit. We are to eat the Word. Jesus said that those who hunger and thirst after righteousness would be filled (Mt. 5:6). The apostle Paul sometimes referred to the Word of God as milk or as meat (1 Cor. 3:2; Heb. 5:12).

If the Bible seems boring or hard to understand, but you want to feed your spirit so you can be healthy, strong, and whole, then ask God to give you a greater hunger for the Word. Actually, we need to give all our desires and appetites to the Lord. Perhaps the hunger that you thought was physical is actually a spiritual hunger. So develop a taste for the things of God. Treat your spiritual man because it is the spiritual man who is hungry.

In John 6:35 Jesus said, "I am the bread of life: he that cometh to Me shall never hunger; and he that believeth on Me shall never thirst." He was comparing Himself to the manna God had sent to feed the children of Israel during their 40-year journey to the Promised Land.

Jesus is like manna from Heaven. If you don't know Him, then you don't know what you are missing. A relationship with the Lord provides the spiritual life and nourishment we all need and crave. Only Jesus can satisfy the hunger of our spirits.

We all know that the body functions best when we feed it healthy foods on a regular basis. The spirit functions best when we "feed" it the food of fellowship with the Lord. As you and I minister to God, He ministers to us. He'll make our hearts, minds, and spirits more vitalized, and that will make a great difference in the life and health of our bodies.

Determine to spend time each day in communication with God. Just as reading the Word is like feeding the spirit, so prayer is like exercising the spirit. Your spirit needs exercise to be healthy just as your body does. Perhaps when you are out for a walk, you can spend that time in prayer. Have a good time with the Lord. Enjoy the fresh air and the beauty of His creation. There are few things like getting out in the wonder of nature to make you appreciate how the Lord has blessed you.

The Bible says, "And truly our fellowship is with the Father, and with His Son Jesus Christ" (1 John 1:3b). Think how a good relationship with your spouse, parent, or close friend ministers to your emotions. When you feel loved, you feel more confident, more capable. A good relationship with God can do even more for you. When assured of God's love and care, you feel as though you can conquer the world—and you can!

The apostle Paul wrote, "I can do all things through Christ which strengtheneth me" (Phil. 4:13). What a tremendous boost to your confidence it is to know that you have a relationship with God. You are one of His children and He is looking out for you. When you have that kind of strength, no diet can defeat you!

Prayer can strengthen you to face temptation and overcome it. When you come up against something that you were not able to handle in the past, this time, breathe a quiet prayer for strength and help from the Lord. It can be a short, simple "prayergram" such as Peter prayed when he found himself about to drown in the Sea of Galilee. "...he cried, saying, Lord, save me. And immediately Jesus stretched forth His hand, and caught him..." (Mt. 14:30-31). There wasn't time for a long theological prayer. All Peter could do was cry out for help. However, that was all it took to bring an immediate answer. The Lord is just as ready and willing to lend you a hand when you have a need.

We all have our moments of need. It isn't a weakness to call out to God for help; it is a strength. Temptations come to all of us and the only sure way to win over them is to draw upon the strength of the Lord.

Food and the Fall

If you find that your biggest temptation is in dealing with food, you are not alone. In fact, the very first temptation to come to mankind wasn't about adultery or murder. The first temptation was to take a bite of forbidden food.

Genesis 2:16 says, "And the Lord God commanded the man, saying, Of every tree of the garden thou mayest freely eat: but of the tree of the knowledge of good and evil, thou shalt not eat of it: for in the day that thou eatest thereof thou shalt surely die."

The death that God spoke of in this verse was a spiritual death. Because of Adam and Eve's sin back in the Garden of Eden, the spirit in each individual must be brought back to life. It was food that caused man to fall.

Genesis 3:1 goes on to tell the story. "Now the serpent was more subtil that any beast of the field...." The word *serpent* means fascinator, tempter. People are fascinated with rich food, nice houses, wads of money, and fast cars. Nothing is wrong with all these things as long as we put them in the right perspective.

Many people are hungry for fame and fortune. They are stepping over one another to get ahead in life. Again, there is nothing wrong with getting ahead, as long as we do it in the right spirit. The Bible says, "Humble yourselves therefore under the mighty hand of God, that He may exalt you in due time" (1 Pet. 5:6).

Many people think it is God who humbles us. It isn't. We humble ourselves before Him and He is the One who exalts us. If we maintain the right spirit, He will help us reach our goals in life.

Most people seem to be fascinated more with the natural things of this life than with the spiritual. People are fascinated with clothes, jewelry, and other luxuries. We can have these things, but we must put first things first. Jesus is "number one." "But seek ye first the kingdom of God, and His righteousness; and all these things shall be added unto you" (Mt. 6:33).

When satan—the serpent—came to Adam and Eve in the garden, his goal was to get their eyes off the spiritual and onto the physical. He said to the woman, "Yea, hath God said, Ye shall not eat of every tree of the garden?" (Gen. 3:1).

Notice that he said "every tree." He was trying to make Eve question God's Word and make her feel as if she were being deprived of something. It's a ploy he still uses today. If you've struggled to deny yourself a piece of pie or a second helping of mashed potatoes, you've experienced this same temptation. The consequences are very different, but the temptation hasn't changed much over the years.

Then the serpent put more doubts in her mind. He said, "...Ye shall not surely die: for God doth know that in the day ye eat thereof, then your eyes shall be opened, and ye shall be as gods, knowing good and evil" (Gen. 3:4-5). Again, the devil was questioning what God had said. In fact, he contradicted the very statement God had made. God had pronounced the consequences of eating the forbidden fruit in no uncertain terms.

What made the risk worth taking to Adam and Eve? Why were they willing to disobey God's commandment? "And when the woman saw that the tree was good for food, and that it was pleasant to the eyes, and a tree to be desired to make one wise, she took of the fruit thereof, and did eat, and gave also unto her husband with her; and he did eat" (Gen. 3:6).

Adam and Eve were in fellowship with the Lord until that time. They were fellowshipping spirit to Spirit, walking in oneness of mind and heart. But they stopped eating of that fellowship. They took their eyes off the words of God and started looking at the fruit, and they fell.

Temptation comes through the eyes and the mind. That's why it is so important that we be careful about the words and images we eat. They have a powerful influence upon us. When we're tempted by food, it appears to be a temptation with only physical consequences. But very often food is such a temptation because we have let our spirits grow weak or weary. We've not fed the inner man well enough to have the strength and inner conviction to resist temptation—any temptation—when it comes.

Adam and Eve tried to substitute physical food and what it could bring them for the spiritual food of fellowshipping with God. It was a poor substitute then, and it still is today.

Submitted to the Lord

If your goal is to be a whole, healthy person rather than to simply take off a few pounds, then you won't downplay the importance of your spirit to your health and wholeness. How can you be the person you want to be if a part of you is dead or sleeping? How can you be strong and confident if you have doubts about your standing with God?

Remember, the devil makes it his business to attack us at our weak points. If cheesecake is our weakness, he won't tempt us with Brussels sprouts. He puts questions in our minds to get us to doubt God. He did it with Adam and Eve, he tried it with Jesus, and he does the same thing with us today. If our spirits are weak, the doubts can undermine every other part of our lives.

The devil tries to get you and I to wonder. We wonder if God cares about us. We wonder if He meant what He said in His Word. Then we wonder if we are living up to His Word. Finally we begin to wonder if living the Christian life isn't just too hard. If we wonder too long and too much, then we start to wander away from our commitment and from God.

Of course, I'm not advocating a super-spirituality that is phoney and contrived. We don't have to walk around polishing our halos or endlessly quoting Scripture. Self-righteousness isn't true spirituality anyway. Humility, graciousness, caring, and love are the true spiritual qualities.

You grow in these and other spiritual qualities by submitting your life to God and committing yourself totally to Him. Settle in your own mind once and for all that you will follow the Lord. Then when the serpent comes along to tempt you, he will find that you aren't so easily confused by his questions.

Faith is a decision, just as love is. You have to decide to love yourself, to love others, and to love

God. You also have to decide to believe God, no matter what the circumstances may be. When you pray for something—even if it is big—don't think, "How will it get done?" Believe it is done when you pray. Don't let your mind wonder and then wander away from faith in God. The Bible says, "But without faith it is impossible to please Him: for he that cometh to God must believe that He is, and that He is a rewarder of them that diligently seek Him" (Heb. 11:6).

Always speak the Word, no matter what situation you are in. You listen to yourself anyway, whether or not you think you do. What you want to hear are words of hope, love, and faith. Those are the words found in the Bible. Speak them and you'll be feeding not only your spirit, but your mind and heart as well.

Early in the morning and late in the evening are the times you are most sensitive to spiritual things. When you get up in the morning, just start praising and worshiping, reading the Word, singing to the Lord, making confessions to Him. Look in the mirror and say, "I am the righteousness of God in Christ Jesus. I desire the Word. I am living a victorious life over temptation and sin. I am gaining control over the problems of my life. I am reaching a healthy weight!" Make your confessions based on what you are believing for, and then watch them become a reality.

Wisdom and Practicality

Remember, though, you don't have to be so heavenly minded that you are no earthly good. We are the light of the world. We are the salt of the earth. We are flesh-and-blood human beings who live in the "here and now" with purpose, commitment, and abundant life.

The life of the spirit is not a mystical thing. It is true that we cannot see with our physical eyes much of what concerns spiritual matters. Therefore, we must accept many things by faith. But the life of the spirit is really very practical. It is a matter of applying the wisdom—and just plain common sense—that God has given us in the Bible.

The Bible is a guidebook that deals with everyday life. It teaches us how to live in such a way that we are healthy, whole, vital, loving, caring people. With strong spirits, fed by God and His Word, we can be our very best.

God doesn't look on the outward appearance of people as the world does. He can look inside us and it is the inner person that He wants to see grow and become strong. If we stay pure in heart and spirit, we will stand righteous before God. Proverbs 10:3 says, "The Lord will not suffer the soul of the righteous to famish: but He casteth away the substance of the wicked."

We need to stay right with God. When you and I say we are faith people, we need to live that out by walking in faith and love. We must take charge of our characters. We must be strong inside. To be spiritual—truly spiritual—is to have the victory over ourselves. That's the greatest victory of all.

Chapter 10

Total Living

Common sense is the knack of seeing things as they are, and doing things as they ought to be done.

—Josh Billings

Balancing the Appetites

We are all very complex creatures. There are no easy answers for the problems and difficulties that we face in life. Each day can hold both promises and problems, both struggles and fulfillment. The people who find the secret of living are whole people who know how to balance all the various parts of their lives.

If we are spiritual, we will have things under control. Those who brag about how spiritual they are usually don't have the physical and mental aspects of their lives under control. They are out of balance. That's why they can only brag on the spiritual things.

It is good to build ourselves up spiritually and to have a strong relationship with God. The importance of that part of our lives cannot be overemphasized. But any truly spiritual person knows that a healthy life includes more than just the spirit. Such a person has balance and control in every area of life.

We can't be spiritual and overeat all the time. If we were spiritual, we would be sensitive to the wisdom of God concerning the care of His temple. After all, the Bible teaches us that the body is the temple not only of our spirit, but of God's Spirit as well. He dwells within us. "Know ye not that ye are the temple of God, and that the Spirit of God dwelleth in you? If any man defile the temple of God, him shall God destroy; for the temple of God is holy, which temple ye are" (1 Cor. 3:16-17).

Many people mistakenly think that God is not concerned about our bodies, and so we needn't be either. They think being spiritual means ignoring the body or beating it into subjection. They see the body, with all its carnal appetites, as evil. But God said our bodies are His dwelling place. He resides within the heart that has invited Him in. Nowhere in the Bible does God advocate mistreating or abusing our bodies. We are to take care of them as we would anything else held precious by the Lord.

Throughout this book we have stressed the need for balance. The needs of the spirit should be balanced with the needs of the body, the mind, and the heart. We are mental, emotional, physical, social, and spiritual beings. If we emphasize one part to the exclusion of the other parts, then we will be off balance.

Perhaps people who eat in excess don't realize it is the spiritual part, not the physical part, that needs food. God will help you find a balance for the appetites. If you eat in excess, God will help you control the hunger for physical food and give you a greater hunger for spiritual food if you ask Him for that help.

Growing as a Christian means learning how to keep your life in balance. Sure, you need to control the appetites of the flesh. Neither can you give in to every craving of the emotions. Self-control is considered one of the fruits of the spirit. It is a product of a life that is growing and becoming more like our Father.

A lack of balance is a subtle imperfection that deceives many people. When they realize they have a problem with their weight, they assume it is a physical problem and look for only physical solutions. But as we have discussed, a weight problem could arise from many different areas. So the best way to find a solution is to take a "whole person" approach.

This approach works not just for weight, but for everything else in your life. Pray for solutions. Listen to your spirit. Examine your thoughts and emotions. Look at your surroundings. What is your life style and how might it be contributing to that problem? In the middle of every problem is the seed of its solution. By approaching life as a whole person, you find whole solutions, not partial ones.

Spirit Versus Flesh

Even the apostle Paul admitted that he sometimes seemed to have a war raging inside him. His spirit wanted to go one way and his flesh wanted to go another. Sometimes it can seem as if we are a bundle of contradictions. The needs and desires of one part of us pulls against the needs and desires of another part of us.

A spirit that has been born anew is one that desires to please God. It is one that seeks integrity, love, commitment, and self-control. But the mind still wants to look for loopholes in the law, and the emotions still demand attention. The body just wants to be fed. How do you reconcile all these different desires and demands battling within you?

The struggle is certainly not a new one. The spiritual and physical parts of us have been warring since Adam and Eve took a bite of the forbidden fruit. Adam and Eve were very spiritual at one time, but then they fell into sin and became very carnal. So we have been struggling with the problem of sin ever since. The Bible is filled with examples of people who fought to be whole and to find the balance between spirit and flesh.

In Genesis 25:27-34 we read a story about a man who made the wrong choice when deciding between spiritual and physical hunger. Esau was a man of the field and a hunter. He was also very carnal and did not value spiritual things. He lived for the moment, never considering the consequences of his actions.

Esau's twin brother Jacob was more spiritual than Esau. Jacob placed a greater value on spiritual matters than Esau did and he had a greater vision for the future because of it. One day Esau came in from an unsuccessful hunt. He was famished and thought he would die if he didn't have a meal.

What crazy, carnal thinking Esau was guilty of. When he saw that his brother Jacob was cooking soup, Esau begged him for some of it. But Jacob put a price on that bowl of soup. He asked for the birthright that entitled Esau to the greater inheritance and the spiritual blessing of their father. Esau knowingly and willingly sold his birthright for a bowl of soup.

Later Esau was to deeply regret that decision and he hated his brother Jacob for it. He claimed that Jacob had tricked him into giving up his rights as the eldest son. But the deal was made out in the open and there was really no trickery involved. Esau simply made a very bad choice. He chose food—one meal—over spiritual and material wealth. He lost so much, including his dignity and self-respect. Jacob wasn't particularly ethical in how he got the birthright, but he did have a better sense of what was truly important in life.

All Esau had to do at that moment of physical hunger was pray to the Lord, "Give me strength." He wouldn't have died from missing one meal or even several meals. The momentary pleasure of a bowl of soup was hardly worth losing his birthright. If his priorities had been different, he might have established the great nation of Israel. Instead, he occupies only a minor role in biblical history.

Many times we try to fight a spiritual warfare in the flesh just as Esau did. We can't do it. The flesh wants what it wants, when it wants it. It is the nature of carnal desires to want immediate gratification, while the spirit knows we have an eternity and can afford to wait.

Esau was carnal. He didn't want to wait to have his physical hunger satisfied. He didn't think of spiritual things—only of the gnawing hunger in his belly. If he had been feeding his spirit, he would not have been controlled by his fleshly desires. Then he would not have lost so much from his life.

You and I are different, though. We are re-created. We are spiritual people. As we seek to be whole and healthy, we know we must give the spiritual part of us more room to grow. We must find the balance between the spirit and the flesh. There must be an involvement of the spirit, the mind, and the emotions in all the decisions we make.

We are not alone in this struggle. In everything we attempt to do in life, we have a Partner. Our heavenly Father can help us with the trials and temptations we face. He can provide us with strength, wisdom, patience, persistence, and whatever else we need to overcome those trials and temptations. God is not concerned just about the spiritual part of us. He wants us to be whole people—balanced, wise, and healthy—living life to the fullest as He intended.

The Little Word NO

Esau lost his birthright for a bowl of soup. Adam and Eve fell from grace in the Garden of Eden for a piece of fruit. Do you know why the children of Israel wanted to go back to Egypt after Moses had led them out of slavery? For the food! (See Numbers 11:4-6.) The devil always tries to draw people back to the carnal, back into the world, back toward giving in to the desires that are neither healthy nor wise.

The devil is a whisperer. He whispers, "Oh, you can have that cheesecake there. It won't hurt just this one time." He whispers, "Go ahead and have a good cry. You've been so mistreated—you deserve to pamper yourself." He whispers, "Everyone else is doing it. What's so bad about a few drinks?"

One of the devil's best tools is making us fear the word *no*. We don't want to say no to ourselves. We feel like deprived martyrs if we deny ourselves something. When the world is not whispering but shouting that everyone should look out for themselves, go for the gusto, and get everything they can, *no* can be a very difficult word to deal with.

Keith was a man who didn't like to say no. So he seldom ever said it to himself. If he wanted something, he went and got it. He wanted a Mercedes; he bought it. He wanted a boat; he bought it. He wanted to be vice-president of the computer company where he worked by the time he was 35; he did whatever he felt it would take to get that position.

Part of his job as vice-president involved entertaining clients and being very active in the social scene of the community. He actually owned two tuxedos because he and his wife Louise were always attending dinners and other social functions.

Keith liked to eat and since he never said no to himself, he ate whatever he wanted, whenever he wanted. It embarrassed Louise that he habitually ate what she left on her plate after a dinner. But she never wanted to say anything until he started eating off of other people's pushed-back plates as well.

One evening they were dressing for another dinner party and Keith complained that the dry cleaners had shrunk his tux. Louise had to bite her tongue to keep from saying it wasn't the suit that had changed sizes. Keith didn't like to be contradicted.

But her concern showed on her face anyway. At his last medical check-up, the doctor had told Keith that his blood pressure was too high and he needed to lose weight. Louise didn't know how she would convince Keith to change his ways.

After dinner, as always, Keith looked at the chocolate cake on Louise's plate and said, "If you're not going to eat that, can I have it?" The Louse did something she had never done before. Quietly, but firmly, she said, "No."

Keith looked as if he had been slapped. What had gotten into Louise? Since they were sharing a table with the company president and the mayor, he didn't pursue it then. But when they got home that evening he asked her about it.

"I've never said anything about your eating off other people's plates," Louise explained, "because it seemed like a small thing. But it really embarrasses me. And it's creating a weight problem for you."

Her words stunned Keith because he had never suspected how Louise felt, or even considered that his actions might be embarrassing to her and detrimental to himself. But because he really did love his wife, he made a decision to change. It was tough, too, because Keith wasn't used to denying himself anything. But with Louise's help, he made some positive improvements in his life.

Overcoming the temptations we face is as simple as developing the ability to say no. The anti-drug campaign in recent years has made "just say no" almost a cliché, but it does work. Of course, no one can say no without an inner strength of purpose and character. Telling someone to just say no is easy, but doing it ourselves is hard. We must have something inside us—strong spirits—to be able to say no.

Keith found that once he made the decision to change some things in his life, his conscience would bother him every time he slipped. That is one way our spirits work with all the other parts of us to help us be our best.

Your conscience may seem like a nag at times. But without a conscience, we would be in trouble very quickly. We need that little voice inside us to steer us in the right direction. The people who have experienced a spiritual rebirth find that the spirit has a wonderful instinctive knowledge of right and wrong. If we listen to it, we make good decisions. If we don't listen to it, we make harmful mistakes.

When you are spiritual, you get strength and wisdom about what to eat and what not to eat. When you are spiritual, you learn how to be a more fulfilled person. When you are spiritual, you develop a healthy self-esteem based upon your understanding of your place in God. When you are spiritual, you grow in your relationships with other people.

Let's Get Spiritual

All those things are influenced by the spiritual part of us because they are taught to us in the Bible—our spiritual guidebook. Those people who say the Bible isn't relevant for today, haven't read it. The Bible is an incredibly practical book, filled with common-sense guidelines for living. Long before doctors told us obesity was a life-threatening problem, the Bible told us that gluttony (overeating) was a sin.

Why is overeating a sin? Some people think God just wants to ruin our fun. That is hardly true. Gluttony is a sin because it hurts us. It is life-threatening. God is trying to help us, not hurt us, when He tells us not to overeat. The same is true for all the other laws and commandments He has given us. They are there for our protection. God wants a good life for us and His Book tells us how we can live such a life.

Study the Book. You'll find answers there to most, if not all, the questions you have about living this life here on earth. The Bible helps you make sense out of things. It helps you establish priorities and develop character. It gives you a practical plan for life.

People who do not read the Bible or follow God don't know the spiritual system of the way things work. Life can seem very confusing and frightening when you have nothing to guide you. Even people sitting in church pews, thinking they are very spiritual for attending services, can be lost because they are not really in tune with their spirits and with God. That's why they eat the wrong things. That's why they listen to the wrong things. That's why they say the wrong things. They don't know how to gain the strength they need in every area of life.

You may be thinking, from what has been said in these last two chapters, that eating is a sin, that it's unspiritual, or that God frowns on our enjoying a good meal. That isn't true.

God provided us with all the food on earth. He also has given us certain guidelines about what is good for us and what isn't. I guess that makes God the first nutritionist. But He has never said that we shouldn't eat or that we shouldn't enjoy the food He created.

The Bible is filled with stories about how God provided His people with food. In Genesis we read about Joseph. God placed him in Egypt at the time of a severe world famine so he could devise a plan to provide food for the people (see Gen. 45:5-7).

When God was leading the children of Israel out of Egypt more than 400 years later, He again provided them with food—manna and quail. The manna never ran out until they reached the Promised Land (Josh. 5:12).

The Bible says Elijah was out in the wilderness feeling sorry for himself. The Lord wanted him to go on a 40-day journey, but Elijah wasn't ready to go. So God sent an angel to bring Elijah food. God knew that Elijah needed to eat something before he could face the difficult journey ahead (1 Kings 19:4-8).

See how practical God is? He doesn't ask you to be a martyr where food is concerned. He simply wants you to use common sense. He wants you to be strong spiritually so you have the ability to say no to the temptations. He wants you to yield your life to Him so He can lead you in the best way for your life.

Remember, it is the spiritual person who needs to be nurtured and brought to life. Once the spiritual part of you has strength, then you will mature. You will be strong and whole. That inner person must be fed so you can feed every other part of you in a healthy way.

As you follow and yield to God, He will guide your every decision—even decisions as small as what to eat or what not to eat. When you become spiritually mature, everything else will be balanced and you'll be healthy and whole.

Chapter 11

The Whole Person

What Have You Learned?

We've covered a lot in this book, and I hope it has been helpful in getting you started on a healthier, happier, and more successful life style. The people who really live life fully are those who learn that they are more than one-dimensional creatures. They pay attention to every area of their lives and find wholeness and satisfaction.

You are a spirit, you live in a physical body, and you relate to the world around you on a mental, emotional, and social level. Any success that you enjoy in life comes as you seek to be healthy and whole in each of these areas. If one part of you is unhealthy, it will eventually create problems for every other part of you.

It's like having a leak in the deepest part of a ship. It may seem harmless to the upper deck, but if that little leak is left unattended, sooner or later it will send the whole ship floundering in the waters. You can bail water for a while and be okay, but if you want to be more than just okay, you must fix the leak.

So roll up your sleeves and put on your working-out shoes. Living a healthy, whole life style takes dedication and hard work. It involves understanding who you are, what you think, what you believe, how you feel, how you act, and how you respond to others. It means applying the lessons you've learned in reading this book.

Let's review here the important points we've discussed. You might want to copy these points and place them in strategic places around your home to daily remind you of what you are learning as you become a whole person. Also, don't forget to put up pictures that feed your mind with positive, healthy images.

Mental

Dieting is a matter of the mind. It requires balance and control to be a whole person and not simply a thin person. Since many of our problems begin in our minds, the solution to those problems must also begin in the mind. Remember:

1. You are what you think because what you think is what you become.

2. Beliefs influence behavior and behavior produces results.
3. Positive, healthy thoughts create positive, healthy people.
4. Identify your negative thoughts and beliefs and then you will be able to change them.
5. You get rid of negative thoughts by replacing them with positive ones.
6. You can overcome the past by putting it behind you.
7. The words you eat should be healthy and positive because you are what you eat.
8. Positive words and images create power and strength in your mind and spirit.
9. By setting new image goals for yourself, you can think your way to a healthier, happier you.
10. The words you speak should reflect and reinforce the positive images and thoughts in your mind.

The power of thoughts and words cannot be underestimated. Therefore you should work to keep your mind healthy and strong by thinking positive thoughts, eating positive words and images, and speaking positive truths. Having a healthy mind is the first step to being a whole, healthy person.

Emotional

Your emotions influence the way you think, the way you talk, and the way you behave. Very little in your life is so dramatic or forceful as your emotions. Positive emotions can pull you up to your highest level and help you become your best. Here are some of the points we covered about emotions:

1. Since your greatest emotional need is to be loved, you must learn to love yourself.
2. Though rejection, disappointment, criticism, insecurity, guilt, and fear are obstacles to loving yourself, these obstacles can be overcome.
3. Many of your emotional responses are simply habits that can be replaced with something more positive.
4. To love yourself and to develop a healthy life style, you must make good choices, maintain healthy attitudes, and exercise the proper control.
5. Making good choices and changes in how you feel will bring good changes in how you behave.
6. You will become a better person when you decide you are worth the effort it takes to change.

7. You must overcome bad attitudes toward yourself if you want to be your best.
8. Negative attitudes are changed at the roots—thoughts and feelings.
9. You must be in control of your thoughts, feelings, and actions rather than surrender control to someone else.
10. Every day that you exercise discipline and control will help you grow stronger.

A diet is only as good as the healthy thoughts and emotions that accompany it. If you can learn to love yourself and make good choices for your life, you can conquer anything.

Physical

Because your body is the most visible part of you, it often becomes the sole focus of attention when it comes to weight loss. Whole people are more than just beautiful bodies, although you can work on improving the physical part of you. Some of the things we covered about the physical aspect of healthy living include the following:

1. You must decide for yourself what weight range you want to reach and maintain.
2. You must let your desires for your health and looks be the factors that determine

your weight goal instead of the pressure to conform to the ideas of others.

3. You can lose all the weight you need to lose if you set realistic goals for short, medium, and long ranges.
4. You change your eating habits by first examining them and recognizing those that are unhealthy.
5. Like your thoughts and attitudes, bad eating habits are changed by replacing them with good ones.
6. You can eat your way to good health and good looks by choosing nutritious, balanced foods.
7. Beauty and strength are qualities that arise from within you and are reflected in your physical appearance.
8. Good looks are a combination of good health and good grooming.
9. Nutritious foods promote beauty as much as they do health.
10. Exercise is a key to fitness, health, and beauty.

Your life style has a very telling effect upon your health and your looks. What you eat, how you work and play, and what your habits and goals are, will all make a difference in your life. You can reach the goal of a healthy, attractive body if you are willing to work at it.

Social

Since food is an important part of most social activities, the social aspect of your life also affects your diet. With the right plan, you can avoid the social traps that stand in the way of your goals. These are the points we covered in our social study:

1. The wide variety and availability of food in society makes it tempting, but you can vanquish that temptation by avoiding the places and situations where you are vulnerable.
2. Traditional and cultural foods can still be enjoyed in moderation and modification.
3. Eating in social settings doesn't have to be hazardous if you follow careful planning and make wise choices.
4. With freedom and strength, you can withstand the pressure to eat and can politely say no to unhealthy foods.
5. Becoming the person you want to be gives you the satisfaction and confidence that makes you a pleasure to be around.
6. Well-established priorities and goals help you withstand social pressures to eat.

7. Your choice of companions influence all the other choices you make in life.
8. Instead of letting your friends determine your desires, you must stand on the convictions of what you know to be right for yourself.
9. Envy and jealousy are a waste of emotional energy and should be replaced with a good feeling about yourself.
10. Being active and involved promotes alertness, positive feelings, and good health.

Making positive changes in yourself takes daring and endurance. It can mean going against peer pressure and making difficult choices. But the result of a healthier, happier you is reward enough for all your efforts.

Spiritual

Your spiritual nature is the most important part of you because it lives on for eternity. Being healthy and strong in your spirit makes a vast difference in how healthy and strong you are in every other part of your life. Here are the points we covered in the spiritual realm:

1. Your spirit is your true self that is brought to new life when you come to God.
2. Spirituality is wisdom and practicality for coping with the challenges of life.

3. Physical food can never satisfy the spiritual hunger that you experience.
4. You feed your spirit through positive words and images from the Word of God.
5. Prayer and communion with the Lord promote growth and strength in your spirit.
6. A relationship with God gives you the confidence that you can conquer the world.
7. If you are strong in your spirit, you can resist the temptation to substitute physical food for spiritual food.
8. Faith is a decision you make, just as love is.
9. With a strong spirit, fed by God and His Word, you can be your best.
10. Growing healthy and strong means keeping all the parts of your life in balance.

Achieving wholeness can sometimes seem like a difficult battle. But you were created to be a whole person and if you are willing to work at reaching that goal, you can be a healthy, happy, successful individual.

No one can tell you what you should weigh. No one can tell you what you should wear, what you should think, or what you should do. These are things you must decide for yourself. Choose to be your very best. Don't settle for anything less than your fullest, God-given potential. He made you and He doesn't intend for His work to go to waste. He desires that you be fulfilled in every area of life. With God on your side, you can't lose. You can be a whole person—starting today.

Ira Kellman is available for ministry in various types of meetings. Ira is a teacher/evangelist who ministers in a simple, clear, and yet profound way. God uses him in the ministry of healings, miracles, and creative miracles. There are results in every meeting.

Ira ministers to singles groups, married couples, business organizations (motivational), professional sports clubs (chapel services, counseling), and in churches, seminars, and crusades.

You can contact him at:

Ira Kellman Ministries
P.O. Box 35187
Tulsa, OK 74153

Phone/FAX: 918-251-4717

Other Products by Ira Kellman

Stirring, anointed cassette tapes by Ira Kellman are also available. Write to the following address to request a list.

Ira Kellman Ministries
P.O. Box 35187
Tulsa, OK 74153